STUDY GUIDE FOR

Lippincott Williams & Wilkins'

ADMINISTRATIVE Medical Assisting

STUDY GUIDE FOR

Lippincott Williams & Wilkins'

ADMINISTRATIVE Medical Assisting

THIRD EDITION

Laura Southard Durham, BS, CMA

Medical Assisting Technologies Program Coordinator (Retired)
Forsyth Technical Community College
Winston-Salem, North Carolina

Wolters Kluwer | Lippincott Williams & Wilkins
Health

Philadelphia • Baltimore • New York • London
Buenos Aires • Hong Kong • Sydney • Tokyo

Acquisitions Editor: Kelley Squazzo
Senior Product Manager: Amy Millholen
Design Coordinator: Stephen Druding
Marketing Manager: Shauna Kelley
Compositor: SPi Global
Printer: RR Donnelley–Shenzhen

351 West Camden Street
Baltimore, MD 21201

Two Commerce Square
2001 Market Street
Philadelphia, PA 19103

Printed in China

ISBN: 9781451115802

To purchase additional copies of this book, call our customer service department at (800) 638-3030 or fax orders to (301) 223-2320. International customers should call (301) 223-2300.

Visit Lippincott Williams & Wilkins on the Internet: http://www.lww.com. Lippincott Williams & Wilkins customer service representatives are available from 8:30 am to 5:00 pm, EST.

13
1 2 3 4 5 6 7 8 9 10

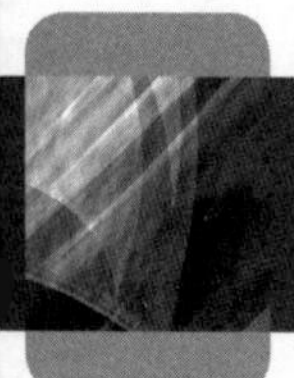

Preface

Welcome to the *Study Guide for Lippincott Williams & Wilkins' Administrative Medical Assisting, Third Edition.* In this edition, we have aligned the exercises and activities with the most current (2008) Medical Assisting Education Review Board (MAERB) of the American Association of Medical Assistants (AAMA) curriculum standards. Program directors, instructors, and students will know which activities in this *Study Guide* support comprehension of knowledge from the textbook (cognitive domain), which support the practice and skills needed to become a competent entry-level medical assistant (psychomotor domain), and which exercises encourage critical thinking and professional behaviors in the medical office (affective domain). This *Study Guide* is unique in a number of ways and offers features that are not found in most Medical Assisting study guides.

The *Study Guide* is divided into sections that coincide with the textbook. Parts I and II include exercises that reinforce the knowledge and skills required of all Medical Assistants. Part III includes activities to "put it all together" as a potential medical office employee.

Each chapter includes the following:

- **Learning Outcomes**—Learning outcomes are listed at the beginning of the chapter and are divided into AAMA/CAAHEP categories (Cognitive, Psychomotor, Affective) and ABHES competencies.
- **A Variety of Question Formats**—To meet the needs of a variety of learning styles and to reinforce content and knowledge, each chapter of the *Study Guide* includes multiple choice, matching, short answer, completion, and where applicable, calculation-type questions. These formats will help you retain new information, reinforce previously learned content, and build confidence.
- **Case Studies for Critical Thinking**—These scenarios and questions are designed with real-world situations in mind and are intended to promote conversation about possible responses, not just one correct answer! These questions will be valuable to students who confront these types of situations during externship and graduates who encounter similar situations after employment.
- **Procedure Skill Sheets**—Every procedure in the textbook has a procedure skill sheet in the *Study Guide.* These procedures have been updated and revised in this edition and include steps on interacting with diverse patients, such as those who are visually or hearing impaired, those who do not speak English or who speak English as a second language (ESL), and patients who may have developmental challenges.
- **Putting it all Together**—Chapter 17 in the *Study Guide* gives students the opportunity to reinforce information learned throughout their program. This final *Study Guide* chapter includes documentation skills practice for a multitude of situations and active learning activities to engage students with previously learned knowledge.

This *Study Guide* has been developed in response to numerous requests from students and instructors for a concise, understandable, and interactive resource that covers the skills necessary to become a successful Medical Assistant. We hope you find the exercises and tools in this book productive and useful towards your goal of becoming the best Medical Assistant possible!

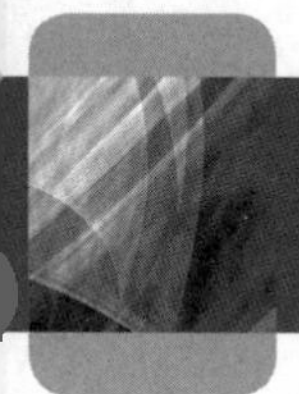

Contents

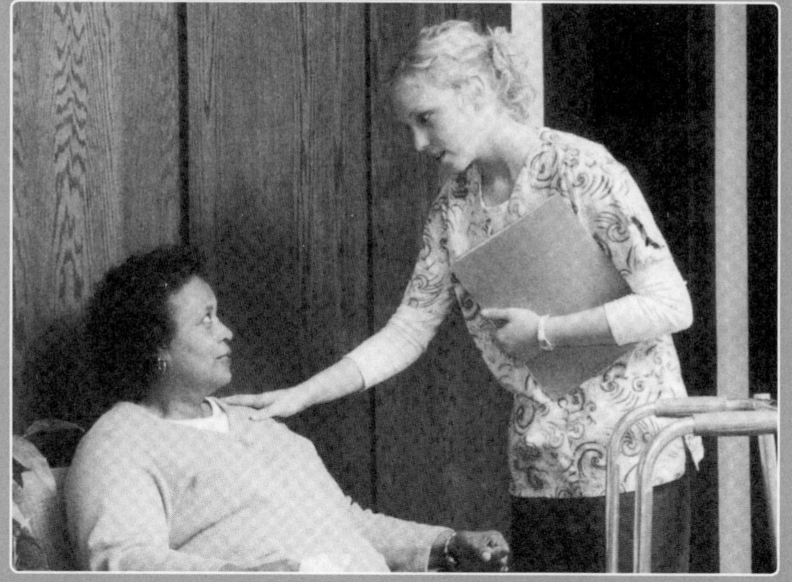

PART

I

Introduction to Medical Assisting

UNIT ONE

Understanding the Profession

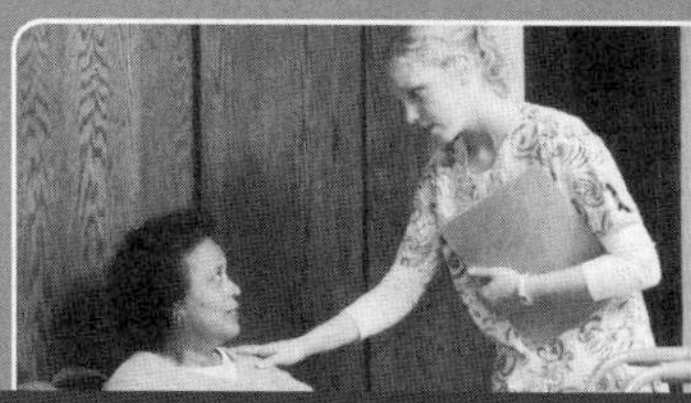

CHAPTER 1

Medicine and Medical Assisting

Learning Outcomes

Cognitive Domain

1. Spell and define the key terms
2. Summarize a brief history of modern medicine
3. Explain the system of health care in the United States
4. Discuss the typical medical office
5. List medical specialties a medical assistant may encounter
6. List settings in which medical assistants may be employed
7. List the duties of a medical assistant
8. Describe the desired characteristics of a medical assistant
9. Discuss legal scope of practice for medical assistants
10. Compare and contrast physician and medical assistant roles in terms of standard of care
11. Recognize the role of patient advocacy in the practice of medical assisting
12. Identify the role of self boundaries in the health care environment
13. Differentiate between adaptive and non-adaptive coping mechanisms
14. Identify members of the health care team
15. Explain the pathways of education for medical assistants
16. Discuss the importance of program accreditation
17. Name and describe the two nationally recognized accrediting agencies for medical assisting education programs
18. Explain the benefits and avenues of certification for the medical assistant
19. Discuss licensure and certification as it applies to health care providers
20. List the benefits of membership in a professional organization
21. Identify the effect peronal ethics may have on professional performance
22. Compare personal, professional, and organizational ethics
23. Discuss all levels of governmental legislation and regulation as they apply to medical assisting practice, including FDA and DEA regulations

Psychomotor Domain

1. Perform within scope of practice
2. Practice within the standard of care for a medical assistant
3. Develop a plan for separation of personal and professional ethics
4. Respond to issues of confidentiality
5. Document accurately in the patient record

Affective Domain

1. Demonstrate awareness of the consequences of not working within the legal scope of practice
2. Apply ethical behaviors, including honesty and integrity in performance of medical assisting practice

3. Examine the impact personal ethics and morals may have on the individual's practice

ABHES Competencies

1. Comprehend the current employment outlook for the medical assistant
2. Compare and contrast the allied health professions and understand their relation to medical assisting
3. Understand medical assistant credentialing requirements and the process to obtain the credential. Comprehend the importance of credentialing
4. Have knowledge of the general responsibilities of the medical assistant
5. Define scope of practice for the medical assistant, and comprehend the conditions for practice within the state that the medical assistant is employed
6. Demonstrate professionalism by:
   a. Exhibiting dependability, punctuality, and a positive work ethic
   b. Exhibiting a positive attitude and a sense of responsibility
   c. Maintaining confidentiality at all times
   d. Being cognizant of ethical boundaries
   e. Exhibiting initiative
   f. Adapting to change
   g. Expressing a responsible attitude
   h. Being courteous and diplomatic
   i. Conducting work within scope of education, training, and ability
7. Comply with federal, state, and local health laws and regulations
8. Analyze the effect of hereditary, cultural, and environmental influences

Name: ______________________ Date: __________ Grade: __________

COG MULTIPLE CHOICE

1. Julia is a student in her last year of a medical assisting program. What must she complete before graduating?
   - a. Certification
   - b. An associate's degree
   - c. An externship
   - d. Curriculum

2. Who is eligible to take the RMA examination? Circle all that apply.
   - a. Medical assistants who have been employed as medical instructors for a minimum of 5 years
   - b. Medical assistants who have been employed in the profession for a minimum of 5 years
   - c. Graduates from ABHES-accredited medical assisting programs
   - d. Graduates from CAAHEP-accredited medical assisting programs

3. Marie and Pierre Curie revolutionized the principles of:
   - a. nursing.
   - b. disease.
   - c. infection.
   - d. physics.
   - e. radioactivity.

4. The medical assistant's role will expand over time because of:
   - a. a growing population.
   - b. the risk of disease and infection.
   - c. advances in medicine and technology.
   - d. a financial boom.
   - e. more effective training programs.

5. What drives the management practices of the outpatient medical facility?
   - a. The desire to compete with other medical facilities
   - b. The need to adhere to government rules and regulations
   - c. The attempt to fit into mainstream medical opinion
   - d. The effort to retain medical employees
   - e. The focus on hiring specialized health care workers

6. Which of the following tasks is the administrative team responsible for in the medical office?
   - a. Physical examinations
   - b. Financial aspects of the practice
   - c. Laboratory test processing
   - d. Minor office surgery
   - e. Drawing blood

7. Which of the following is a clinical duty?
   - a. Scheduling appointments
   - b. Obtaining medical histories
   - c. Handling telephone calls
   - d. Filing insurance forms
   - e. Implementing ICD-9 and CPT coding for insurance claims

8. Empathy is the ability to:
   - a. care deeply for the health and welfare of patients.
   - b. keep your temper in check.
   - c. show all patients good manners.
   - d. remain calm in an emergency.
   - e. feel pity for sick patients.

9. If a patient refers to you as a "nurse," you should:
   a. call the physician.
   b. ignore the mistake.
   c. politely correct him or her.
   d. send him or her home.
   e. ask the nurse to come into the room.

10. A group of specialized people who are brought together to meet the needs of the patient is called:
   a. multiskilled.
   b. multifaceted.
   c. multitasked.
   d. multidisciplinary.
   e. multitrained.

11. A medical assistant falls into the category of:
   a. nurse.
   b. physician assistant.
   c. medical office manager.
   d. allied health professional.
   e. all of the above.

12. The discovery of which vaccine opened the door to an emphasis on preventing disease rather than simply trying to cure preventable illnesses?
   a. Smallpox
   b. Cowpox
   c. Puerperal fever
   d. Typhoid
   e. Influenza

13. "Scope of practice" refers to:
   a. the tasks a person is trained to do.
   b. the tasks an employer allows an employee to perform.
   c. limitations placed on employees by law.
   d. a concept that varies from state to state.
   e. all of the above.

14. All accredited programs must include a(n):
   a. medical terminology course.
   b. computer course.
   c. externship.
   d. certification examination.
   e. multidisciplinary program.

15. What is the requirement for admission to the CMA examination?
   a. Successful completion of 60 CEUs
   b. Successful completion of an externship
   c. Graduation from high school
   d. Graduation from an accredited medical assisting program
   e. Successful completion of a GED program

16. An oncologist diagnoses and treats:
   a. disorders of the musculoskeletal system.
   b. disorders of the ear, nose, and throat.
   c. pregnant women.
   d. the aging population.
   e. benign and malignant tumors.

17. A CMA is required to recertify every:
   a. 1 year.
   b. 2 years.
   c. 5 years.
   d. 10 years.
   e. 15 years.

18. Which organization offers the RMA examination?
   a. American Medical Technologists
   b. American Association of Medical Assistants
   c. American Academy of Professional Coders
   d. American Health Information Management Association
   e. American Board of Medical Specialties

19. Which of the following is a benefit of association membership?

a. Time off from work
b. Networking opportunities
c. Hotel expenses
d. Free health insurance
e. Externship placement

20. Which specialist diagnoses and treats disorders of the stomach and intestines?

a. Endocrinologist
b. Gastroenterologist
c. Gerontologist
d. Podiatrist
e. Internist

21. A goal of regenerative medicine is to:

a. replace the need for organ donation.
b. slow the healing process.
c. provide more health care jobs.
d. sell organs commercially.
e. win the Nobel Prize in the medicine category.

22. "Standard of care" refers to:

a. the focus of medicine.
b. generally accepted guidelines and principles that health care practitioners follow in the practice of medicine.
c. a physician's specialty.
d. a concept that only applies to physicians.
e. a policy that was written by Hippocrates.

COG MATCHING

Grade: _______________

Match the following key terms to their definitions.

Key Terms

23. _____ caduceus
24. _____ medical assistant
25. _____ outpatient
26. _____ specialty
27. _____ clinical
28. _____ administrative
29. _____ laboratory
30. _____ multidisciplinary
31. _____ inpatient
32. _____ externship

Definitions

a. completed by a CMA every 5 years by either taking the examination again or by acquiring 60 CEU
b. describing a medical facility where patients receive care but are not admitted overnight
c. a subcategory of medicine that a physician chooses to practice upon graduation from medical school
d. referring to a team of specialized professionals who are brought together to meet the needs of the patient
e. regarding a medical facility that treats patients and keeps them overnight, often accompanied by surgery or other procedure
f. a medical symbol showing a wand or staff with two serpents coiled around it

33. _____ accreditation

34. _____ certification

35. _____ recertification

g. voluntary process that involves a testing procedure to prove an individual's baseline competency in a particular area

h. regarding tasks that involve direct patient care

i. an educational course during which the student works in the field gaining hands-on experience

j. a multiskilled health care professional who performs a variety of tasks in a medical setting

k. a nongovernmental professional peer review process that provides technical assistance and evaluates educational programs for quality based on pre-established academic and administrative standards

l. regarding tasks that involve scientific testing

m. regarding tasks that focus on office procedures

COG SHORT ANSWER

Grade: _____

36. What is the purpose of the Centers for Medicare and Medicaid Services?

_____

_____

_____

37. The following are three specialists who may employ medical assistants. Describe what each does.

a. allergist: _____

b. internist: _____

c. gynecologist: _____

COG IDENTIFICATION

Grade: ________

As a medical assistant, you must be "multiskilled," or skilled at completing many different tasks. Almost all the tasks you will complete fall into one of two categories: administrative and clinical. But what's the difference between administrative and clinical tasks? Read each selection below and determine whether the task requires your clinical or administrative skills, then place a C or an A beside the task.

38. _____ preparing patients for examinations

39. _____ maintaining medical records

40. _____ ensuring good public relations

41. _____ obtaining medical histories

42. _____ preparing and sterilizing instruments

43. _____ screening sales representatives

AFF SHORT ANSWER

Grade: ________

44. What qualities do you possess that would make you a valuable member of your professional organization?

____

____

____

45. List the characteristics that you possess that will make you a successful medical assistant.

____

____

____

46. List any personal characteristics you believe you could improve.

____

____

____

47. Describe the personal appearance of a professional medical assistant.

48. What are the two accrediting bodies for the medical assisting education arena?

49. What is the importance of having adaptive coping mechanisms in place? Give an example of a situation in which such tools would be helpful.

50. How would you answer the question, "Legally, who is responsible for the actions of CMAs or RMAs as they perform their skills?"

51. You are a CMA in a busy Ob/Gyn practice. You have been asked to orient a high school student who was hired to help up front and in medical records in the afternoons. She wants a career in health care but is unsure if she would be happier in a doctor's office or a hospital. She is debating between becoming a CMA or a CNA but is confused about the difference. She asks for your help in deciding what profession to choose. How would you explain the difference in the two careers?

52. Why is the ability to respect patient confidentiality essential to the role of the medical assistant?

53. The medical office in which you work treats a variety of patients, from all ages and backgrounds. Why should you work with a multidisciplinary health care team? What are the benefits to the patients?

WHAT WOULD YOU DO?

Grade: ________

54. You are preparing a patient for her examination, but the physician is running behind schedule. The patient is becoming anxious and asks you to perform the examination, instead of the physician. You tell her that you will go check how much longer the physician will be. But she responds, "Can't you just perform the exam? Aren't you like a nurse?" How should you respond?

55. The patient who asked you to perform the examination now refuses to wait for the physician. Even though she has a serious heart condition requiring monthly checkups, she leaves without being treated by the physician. You need to write a note that will be included in her chart and in an incident report. What would you say?

COG AFF PSY ACTIVE LEARNING

Grade: _______

56. Review the list of specialists who employ medical assistants in textbook Table 1-2. Choose one specialty that interests you. Perform research on what kinds of procedures the specialist performs. Then consider what kinds of tasks a medical assistant employed by this specialist might perform. Write a letter to this specialist explaining why you would want to work in this kind of office. Be sure to include specific references to the tasks and procedures that interest you based on your research.

____

____

____

57. Scope of practice for medical assistants can vary from state to state. In some states, CMAs are not allowed to perform invasive procedures, such as injections or phlebotomy. Go to the Web site for your state and research the laws in your state regarding the medical assistant's scope of practice. Why is it important to understand your scope of practice before beginning work in a new medical office?

____

____

____

AFF CASE STUDY FOR CRITICAL THINKING A

Grade: _______

You are a CMA in a family practice where many of your friends and neighbors are patients. One of them is being treated for breast cancer. It seems as though everywhere you go, someone asks about her condition. They are just concerned, and so are you. You really want to give them an update on her treatment, but you know that is prohibited.

58. What is your best action? Choose all appropriate actions from the list below.

a. Ask the patient if she minds letting you give updates to their mutual friends.

b. Tell them that you would be violating a federal law if you discuss her care, but they should call her to find out.

c. Tell them what they want to know. After all, they are asking because they care.

d. Offer to help your friend/patient join a Web site that will allow her to update her friends.

AFF CASE STUDY FOR CRITICAL THINKING B

Grade: __________

You start your new position as a CMA for a busy pediatric practice. You are unsure of your job responsibilities, but the office manager expects you to "hit the ground running." Your first day is busy, and you are asked to handle the phones. Your first caller is a mother who is worried about her child's fever.

59. Your best response is:

- **a.** Don't worry. I'm sure she will be fine.
- **b.** Let me check the office protocol for children with fever. I will call you back.
- **c.** Today is my first day; I don't know, but I think she will be fine.
- **d.** You will need to make an appointment.
- **e.** I'll put you through to the doctor immediately.

60. What action could have prevented this uncomfortable situation?

- **a.** Having the opportunity to observe the office for a few weeks before starting
- **b.** Having read the policy and procedure manual before starting work
- **c.** Having more experience in the medical assisting field
- **d.** Paying better attention in class
- **e.** Refusing to answer the phone

61. You ask another CMA what you should do, and her response is, "I thought you were a CMA; you should know what to do." What is your next best action?

- **a.** Go immediately to your supervisor for guidance.
- **b.** Tell another co-worker what she said and ask what she thinks you should do.
- **c.** Start looking for another job.
- **d.** Tell her that if the facility had trained you properly, you would have known what to do.
- **e.** Tell her that you are doing your best, and you are sure you will get up to speed soon.

AFF CASE STUDY FOR CRITICAL THINKING C

Grade: _____

Mrs. Esposito approaches Jan, a medical assistant, at the front desk. Jan has recently treated Mrs. Esposito's son, Manuel, for a foot injury. Mrs. Esposito has just arrived in the United States and, with broken English, asks Jan if she may have her son's medical records to show Manuel's soccer coach that he will be unable to play for the rest of the season. Jan tries to explain to Mrs. Esposito that because her son is 18 years old and legally an adult, she must have his permission to release his medical records. Mrs. Esposito is frustrated and angry. Using Spanish translating software, Jan calmly attempts to explain that the physician would be happy to write a note for Manuel to give to his soccer coach explaining his injuries. After a great deal of time and effort, Mrs. Esposito thanks her for this information and apologizes for becoming angry.

62. From the list below, choose the characteristic of a professional medical assistant that Jan exhibited in the above scenario.

a. Accuracy

b. Proper hygiene

c. The ability to respect patient confidentiality

d. Honesty

63. What was the best action for Jan when she learned that Mrs. Esposito did not speak much English?

a. Look in the Yellow Pages for a translator

b. Try to find a Spanish translating software online

c. Enlist the assistance of a fellow employee who speaks fluent Spanish

d. Tell Mrs. Esposito to come back when she can bring a translator

64. When dealing with an angry person such as Mrs. Esposito, the most important action is to:

a. Raise your voice so she will hear you

b. Treat her as she is treating you

c. Remain calm

d. Notify the office manager of a problem

65. When responding to a request for the release of medical information, your first action should be to:

a. explain the policy to the patient

b. check for the patient's signed authorization

c. ask the physician

d. copy the records

CHAPTER

2 Law and Ethics

Learning Outcomes

Cognitive Domain

1. Spell and define the key terms
2. Discuss all levels of governmental legislation and regulation as they apply to medical assisting practice, including the Food and Drug Administration and the Drug Enforcement Agency
3. Compare criminal and civil law as it applies to the practicing medical assistant
4. Provide an example of tort law as it would apply to a medical assistant
5. List the elements and types of contractual agreements and describe the difference in implied and express contracts
6. List four items that must be included in a contract termination or withdrawal letter
7. List six items that must be included in an informed consent form and explain who may sign consent forms
8. List five legally required disclosures that must be reported to specified authorities
9. Describe the four elements that must be proven in a medical legal suit
10. Describe four possible defenses against litigation for the medical professional
11. Explain the theory of respondeat superior, or law of agency, and how it applies to the medical assistant
12. Outline the laws regarding employment and safety issues in the medical office
13. Identify how the Americans with Disabilties Act applies to the medical assisting profession
14. Differentiate between legal, ethical and moral issues affecting health care
15. Explain how the following impact the medical assistant's practice and give examples
    a. Negligence
    b. Malpractice
    c. Statute of limitations
    d. Good Samaritan Act
    e. Uniform Anatomical Gift Act
    f. Living will/advanced directives
    g. Medical durable power of attorney
16. List the seven American Medical Association principles of ethics
17. List the five ethical principles of ethical and moral conduct outlined by the American Association of Medical Assistants
18. Recognize the role of patient advocacy in the practice of medical assisting
19. Describe the purpose of the Self-Determination Act
20. Explore issue of confidentiality as it applies to the medical assistant
21. Describe the implications of the Health Insurance Portability and Accountability Act for the medical assistant in various medical settings
22. Summarize the Patients' Bill of Rights
23. Discuss licensure and certification as it applies to health care providers
24. Describe liability, professional, personal injury, and third party insurance

Psychomotor Domain

1. Monitor federal and state health care legislation (Procedure 2-1)
2. Incorporate the Patients' Bill of Rights into personal practice and medical office policies and procedures
3. Apply local, state, and federal health care legislation and regulation appropriate to the medical assisting practice setting

Affective Domain

1. Demonstrate sensitivity to patient rights
2. Recognize the importance of local, state, and federal legislation and regulations in the practice setting

ABHES Competencies

1. Comply with federal, state, and local health laws and regulations
2. Institute federal and state guidelines when releasing medical records or information
3. Follow established policies when initiating or terminating medical treatment
4. Understand the importance of maintaining liability coverage once employed in the industry

Name: ________________________ Date: __________ Grade: __________

COG MULTIPLE CHOICE

1. The branch of law concerned with issues of citizen welfare and safety is:

   a. private law.
   b. criminal law.
   c. constitutional law.
   d. administrative law.
   e. civil law.

2. Which branch of law covers injuries suffered because of another person's wrongdoings resulting from a breach of legal duty?

   a. Tort law
   b. Contract law
   c. Property law
   d. Commercial law
   e. Administrative law

3. Choose all of the true statements below regarding the Drug Enforcement Agency (DEA).

   a. The DEA regulates the sale and use of drugs.
   b. The DEA regulates the quality of drugs made in the United States.
   c. Providers who prescribe and/or dispense drugs are required to register with the DEA.
   d. Physicians must report inventory of narcotic medications on hand every month to the DEA.
   e. The DEA is a branch of the Department of Justice.
   f. Drug laws are federal and do not vary from state to state.

4. The Health Insurance Portability and Accountability Act of 1996 deals with the patient's right to:

   a. privacy.
   b. choose a physician.
   c. get information prior to a treatment.
   d. interrupt a treatment considered disadvantageous.
   e. refuse treatment.

5. Which of the following can lead a patient to file a suit for abandonment against a physician?

   a. The physician verbally asks to end the relationship with the patient.
   b. A suitable substitute is not available for care after termination of the contract.
   c. The patient disagrees with the reasons given by the physician for the termination.
   d. Termination happens 35 days after the physician's withdrawal letter is received.
   e. The physician transfers the patient's medical records to another physician of the patient's choice.

Scenario for questions 6 and 7: A man is found lying unconscious outside the physician's office. You alert several colleagues, who go outside to assess the man's condition. It is clear that he will be unable to sign a consent form for treatment.

6. How should the physician handle the unconscious man?

   a. Implied consent should be used until the man can give informed consent.
   b. A health care surrogate should be solicited to provide informed consent.
   c. The hospital administration should evaluate the situation and give consent.
   d. The physician should proceed with no-risk procedures until informed consent is given.
   e. The physician should wait for a friend or family member to give consent on the patient's behalf.

7. Once the man wakes up and gives his express consent to a treatment, this implies that he:

   a. no longer needs assistance.
   b. verbally agrees in front of witnesses on an emergency treatment.
   c. authorizes the physician to exchange the patient's information with other physicians.
   d. trusts the physician with emergency procedures that can be deemed necessary at a later time.
   e. is now familiar with the possible risks of the procedure.

8. A diagnosis of cancer must be reported to the Department of Health and Human Services to:

   a. alert the closest family members.
   b. protect the patient's right to treatment.
   c. investigate possible carcinogens in the environment.
   d. check coverage options with the insurance company.
   e. provide research for a national study.

9. What is the difference between licensure and certification?

   a. Licensure is accessible to medical assistants.
   b. Certification standards are recognized nationally.
   c. Licensure indicates education requirements are met.
   d. Certification limits the scope of activity of a physician.
   e. Licensure allows a professional to practice in any state.

10. The Good Samaritan Act covers:

   a. emergency care provided by a medical assistant.
   b. compensated emergency care outside the formal practice.
   c. sensible emergency practice administered outside the office.
   d. emergency practice administered in the hospital to uninsured patients.
   e. emergency care administered in the physician's office before the patient is registered.

11. The term *malfeasance* refers to:

   a. failure to administer treatment in time.
   b. administration of inappropriate treatment.
   c. administration of treatment performed incorrectly.
   d. failure to administer treatment in the best possible conditions.
   e. the physical touching of a patient without consent.

12. Which tort pertains to care administered without the patient's consent?

   a. Duress
   b. Assault
   c. Tort of outrage
   d. Undue influence
   e. Invasion of privacy

13. The statute of limitation indicates:

   a. the privacy rights of a minor receiving care.
   b. the risks that are presented to a patient before treatment.
   c. the responsibilities of a physician toward his or her patients.
   d. the right of a physician to have another physician care for his or her patients while out of the office.
   e. the time span during which a patient can file a suit against a caregiver.

14. The court may assess contributory negligence when a:

   a. team of physicians incorrectly diagnoses the patient.
   b. physician's malpractice is aggravated by the patient.
   c. patient does not follow the physician's prescribed treatment properly.
   d. patient gives inaccurate information that leads to wrong treatment.
   e. physician is entirely responsible for the patient's injury.

15. Which of these best describes the principle of patient advocacy?

   a. A medical assistant must adhere to his or her own code of conduct.
   b. A medical assistant must act first and foremost in the interest of the patient.
   c. A medical assistant must make sure the patient's information remains confidential.
   d. A medical assistant must make sure to act as a mediator between the physician and the patient.
   e. A medical assistant should only perform procedures that agree with his personal ethics.

16. Which of these is the basic principle of bioethics?

a. All patients are entitled to the best possible treatment.

b. Moral issues must be evaluated according to the patient's specific circumstances.

c. Members of the medical community should never compromise their religious beliefs.

d. The medical community must agree on a code of moral standards to apply to controversial cases.

e. Moral issues are guidelines that the medical community is legally bound to follow.

17. What is the American Medical Association's regulation on artificial insemination?

a. Both husband and wife must agree to the procedure.

b. The donor has the right to contact the couple after the child is born.

c. The procedure can only be performed legally in certain states.

d. A donor can be selected only after the husband has tried the procedure unsuccessfully.

e. The couple requesting the procedure has the right to gain information about possible donors.

18. What does the Self-Determination Act of 1991 establish?

a. The physician has the last word on interruption of treatment.

b. A person has the right to make end-of-life decisions in advance.

c. The physician must follow advance directives from a patient verbatim.

d. Family members cannot make decisions about terminating a patient's treatment.

e. If a patient cannot make his or her own decision, a close family member can do so on his or her behalf.

19. Which of these patients would be unable to sign a consent form?

a. A 17-year-old patient requesting information about a sexually transmitted disease

b. A pregnant 15-year-old patient

c. A 16-year-old boy who works full time

d. A 17-year-old girl who requires knee surgery

e. A married 21-year-old patient

20. In a comparative negligence case, how are damages awarded?

a. The plaintiff receives damages based on a percentage of their contribution to the negligence.

b. The defendant does not have to pay the plaintiff anything.

c. The plaintiff and defendant share 50% of the court costs and receive no damages.

d. The plaintiff has to pay damages to the defendant for defamation of character.

e. The plaintiff receives 100% of the damages awarded.

21. Which of these laws protects you from exposure to bloodborne pathogens and other body fluids in the workplace?

a. Civil Rights Act of 1964

b. Self-Determination Act of 1991

c. Occupational Safety and Health Act

d. Americans with Disabilities Act

e. Clinical Laboratory Improvement Act

22. The Food and Drug Administration is:

a. not affiliated with the federal government.

b. regulated by the Department of Health, Education and Welfare.

c. regulates the manufacture, sale and distribution of drugs in the United States.

d. not charged with assessing quality in the manufacture of drugs.

e. divided among states.

COG MATCHING

Grade: _______

Match the following key terms to their definitions.

Key Terms

23. _____ abandonment
24. _____ slander
25. _____ assault
26. _____ battery
27. _____ ethics
28. _____ tort law
29. _____ civil law
30. _____ common law
31. _____ defamation of character
32. _____ defendant
33. _____ deposition
34. _____ durable power of attorney
35. _____ emancipated minor
36. _____ fee splitting
37. _____ fraud
38. _____ libel
39. _____ litigation
40. _____ locum tenens
41. _____ malpractice
42. _____ negligence
43. _____ plaintiff
44. _____ precedents
45. _____ res ipsa loquitur
46. _____ res judicata
47. _____ respondeat superior
48. _____ stare decisis

Definitions

a. a deceitful act with the intention to conceal the truth
b. process of filing or contesting a lawsuit
c. traditional laws outlined in the Constitution
d. a theory meaning that the previous decision stands
e. a person under the age of majority but married or self-supporting
f. previous court decisions
g. a branch of law that focuses on issues between private citizens
h. governs the righting of wrongs suffered as a result of another person's wrongdoing
i. a substitute physician
j. an arrangement that gives the patient's representative the ability to make health care decisions for the patient
k. sharing fees for the referral of patients to certain colleagues
l. the accuser in a lawsuit
m. failure to take reasonable precautions to prevent harm to a patient
n. the accused party in a lawsuit
o. a doctrine meaning "the thing speaks for itself"
p. the unauthorized attempt to threaten or touch another person without consent
q. the physical touching of a patient without consent
r. malicious or false statements about a person's character or reputation
s. written statements that damage a person's character or reputation
t. a process in which one party questions another party under oath
u. an action by a professional health care worker that harms a patient
v. a doctrine meaning "the thing has been decided"
w. a doctrine meaning "let the master answer," also known as the *law of agency*
x. guidelines specifying right or wrong that are enforced by peer review and professional organizations
y. withdrawal by a physician from a contractual relationship with a patient without proper notification
z. oral statements that damage a person's character or reputation

SHORT ANSWER

Grade: _______

49. List six items that must be included in an informed consent form and explain who may sign consent forms.

50. List five legally required disclosures that must be reported to specified authorities.

51. List nine principles cited in the American Medical Association's principles of ethics.

52. List the five ethical principles of ethical and moral conduct outlined by the American Association of Medical Assistants.

COG IDENTIFICATION

Grade: _______________

The Americans with Disabilities Act (ADA) prohibits discrimination against people with disabilities in employment practice. Take a look at the scenarios in this chart and assess whether or not the ADA is being followed correctly. Place a check mark in the appropriate box.

Scenario	ADA-Compliance	ADA-Noncompliance
53. A physician's office extends an offer of employment to a man in a wheelchair but says that due to a shortage of parking, the office cannot offer him a parking space in the garage.		
54. A 46-year-old woman is refused a position on the basis that she is HIV positive.		
55. A mentally ill man with a history of violence is refused a job in a busy office.		
56. A small office with 10 employees chooses a healthy woman over a disabled woman because the office cannot afford to adapt the facilities in the workplace.		
57. A patient's wheelchair-bound husband cannot accompany her to her physician's visits because there is no handicap entrance for visitors.		
58. A job applicant with a severe speech impediment is rejected for a position as an emergency room receptionist.		

Some situations require a report to be filed with the Department of Health with or without the patient's consent. Read the scenarios in the chart below and decide which ones are legally required disclosures.

Scenario	Legally Required Disclosure	No Action Needed
59. A 35-year-old woman gives birth to a healthy baby girl.		
60. A physician diagnoses a patient with meningococcal meningitis.		
61. A 43-year-old man falls off a ladder and breaks his leg. He spends 3 weeks in the hospital.		
62. A teenager is involved in a hit-and-run accident. He is rushed to the hospital, but dies the next day.		
63. A 2-year-old girl is diagnosed with measles.		
64. A man is diagnosed with a sexually transmitted disease and asks the physician to keep the information confidential.		
65. A woman visits the physician's office and tells him she has mumps, but when he examines her, he discovers it is influenza.		

COG IDENTIFICATION

Grade: ____________

66. Which of the following must be included in a patient consent form? Circle all that apply.

  a. Name of the physician performing the procedure
  b. Alternatives to the procedure and their risks
  c. Date the procedure will take place
  d. Probable effect on the patient's condition if the procedure is not performed
  e. Potential risks from the procedure
  f. Patient's next of kin
  g. Any exclusions that the patient requests
  h. Success rate of the procedure

67. Dr. Janeway has decided to terminate his patient, Mrs. King. The office manager drafted the following letter to Mrs. King. However, when you review the letter, you find that there are errors. Read the letter below and then explain the three problems with this letter in the space below.

Dear Mrs. King,

Because you have consistently refused to follow the dietary restrictions and to take the medication necessary to control your high blood pressure, I feel I am no longer able to provide your medical care. This termination is effective immediately.

Because you do not seem to take your medical condition seriously, I'm not sure that any other physician would want to treat you either. I will hold on to your medical records for 30 days and then they will be destroyed.

Sincerely,
Anthony Janeway, MD

a. ____

b. ____

c. ____

ACTIVE LEARNING

68. Research two recent medical malpractice cases on the Internet. Write a brief outline of each case and make a record of whether the tort was intentional or unintentional, and what the outcome of the case was. Compare the cases to see if there is a common theme.

69. Visit a physician's office and make a list of steps that have been taken to comply with the law. For example, if the physician charges for canceling appointments without notice, there is probably a sign by the reception desk to warn patients of the fee. How many other legal requirements can you find? Are there any that are missing?

70. As technology develops, new laws have to be written to protect the rights of patients who use it. Stem cell research is a particularly gray area and has raised many interesting ethical dilemmas. Research some recent legal cases regarding stem cell research, and write a report on some of the ethical issues the cases have raised.

71. You are a medical assistant in a busy office, and the physician has been called away on an emergency. Some of the patients have been waiting for over 2 hours, and one of them urgently needs a physical checkup for a job application. Although you are not officially qualified, you feel confident that you are able to carry out the examination by yourself. Six months later, the patient files a malpractice suit because you failed to notice a lump in her throat that turned out to be cancerous. Describe the law of agency and explain whether it would help you in the lawsuit.

AFF WHAT WOULD YOU DO?

Grade: ___________

72. A family member calls to inquire about a patient's condition. You know that the patient has not given written consent for information to be passed on, but you recognize the person's voice and remember that she came in with the patient the previous day. Explain what you would say and why.

____

____

____

____

COG IDENTIFICATION

Grade: ___________

73. Mrs. Stevens visits Dr. Johnson's office with neck pain. Dr. Johnson examines her and recommends that she see a specialist. Several months later, Mrs. Stevens sues Dr. Johnson for malpractice, claiming that when he examined her, he made her neck pain worse. In court, she provides pictures of her neck that show severe bruising. A specialist confirms that muscle damage has restricted Mrs. Stevens from going about her daily life. Which of the four elements needed in a medical lawsuit has Mrs. Stevens failed to prove? Circle all that apply.

   a. Duty

   b. Dereliction of duty

   c. Direct cause

   d. Damage

AFF PATIENT EDUCATION

Grade: ___________

74. You have a patient who has just been diagnosed with a sexually transmitted disease. After the physician leaves the office, the patient turns to you and begs you to keep the information confidential. It is obvious that the patient is worried and embarrassed. Explain how you would inform the patient about legally required disclosures and what you would say.

____

____

____

____

AFF CASE STUDY FOR CRITICAL THINKING A

Grade: ____________

Pamela Dorsett is a patient at Highland Oaks Family Practice. She is a 40-year-old woman who has five children and a house full of cats. She brings her children in for immunizations, but otherwise you rarely see them. She walks into the office on a busy Monday morning with all five children. They are surrounded by a pungent smell of cat feces. The children are dirty and it appears are being neglected. All five of them have runny noses. She wants the doctor to see them now because she has transportation problems. You are the receptionist that day. Remember, pick the BEST answer.

75. The doctor is legally obligated to see the children at some point because:

- **a.** the children look neglected.
- **b.** there is a legal contract in place.
- **c.** medical ethics dictate it.
- **d.** all of the above.

76. If child neglect is suspected, the physician is required by federal law to:

- **a.** talk to the mother about her care.
- **b.** try to contact a family member.
- **c.** do nothing, as mandated by HIPAA.
- **d.** report the suspicions to authorities.

77. What would your first action be?

- **a.** Try to work the five children into the busy schedule.
- **b.** Consult with the providers.
- **c.** Make future appointments as soon as possible.
- **d.** Have them wait until the end of the day after all scheduled patients have been seen.

COG AFF CASE STUDY FOR CRITICAL THINKING B

Grade: ___________

As a medical assistant, you will be involved in some administrative issues. Read the following scenarios and assess whether the American Medical Association standards for office management are being met. Place a check mark in the appropriate box.

Scenario	Standards Met	Standards Not Met
78. Dr. Benson tells his medical assistant to cancel Mrs. Burke's tests because she recently lost her job and will be unable to pay for them.		
79. Mr. Grant canceled his appointment with less than 24 hours' notice. He was charged a fee as noted in a sign by the receptionist's desk.		
80. Mrs. O'Malley asks Dr. Jones to help her fill out an insurance form. The form is a four-page document that takes Dr. Jones an hour to fill out. Dr. Jones charges Mrs. O'Malley $15 for filling out the form.		
81. Dr. Harris dies suddenly, and his staff tell patients that the office will close and that copies of their medical records will be transferred to another physician.		
82. Mr. Davies owes the physician's office several thousand dollars. He is moving and asks the office to transfer his medical records to his new physician. The office refuses on the grounds that Mr. Davies has not paid his bill.		
83. Mrs. Jones comes into the office for a vaccination. The physician tells the medical assistant to charge her $10 less than other patients because she is elderly and cannot afford the standard charges.		

PSY PROCEDURE 2-1 Monitoring Federal and State Regulations, Changes, and Updates

Name: _______________ Date: __________ Time: __________ Grade: __________

EQUIPMENT: Computer, Internet connection, search engine or Web site list

KEY: 4 = Satisfactory 0 = Unsatisfactory NA = This step is not counted

PROCEDURE STEPS	SELF	PARTNER	INSTRUCTOR
1. Using a search engine, go to the homepage for your state government (Example: http://www.nc.gov) and/or other related sites such as: Centers for Disease Control and Prevention (CDC), Occupational Safety and Health Act (OSHA), your state medical society, and the American Medical Association (AMA).	☐	☐	☐
2. Input keywords such as: Health care finances, allied health professionals, outpatient medical care, Medicare, etc.	☐	☐	☐
3. Create and enforce a policy for timely dissemination of information received by fax or e-mail from outside agencies.	☐	☐	☐
4. Circulate information gathered to all appropriate employees with an avenue for sharing information. Any information obtained should be shared.	☐	☐	☐
5. Post changes in policies and procedures in a designated area of the office.	☐	☐	☐
6. AFF Explain what you would say to a fellow employee who responds to a change in a current law with, "I will just keep doing it the old way. Who is going to care?"	☐	☐	☐

____

____

____

____

CALCULATION

Total Possible Points: _______

Total Points Earned: _________ Multiplied by 100 = _________ Divided by Total Possible Points = _________ %

PASS **FAIL** **COMMENTS:**

☐ ☐

Student's signature _______________________________________ Date _________

Partner's signature _______________________________________ Date _________

Instructor's signature _____________________________________ Date _________

CHAPTER

3 Communication Skills

Learning Outcomes

Cognitive Domain

1. Spell and define the key terms
2. List two major forms of communication
3. Identify styles and types of verbal communication
4. Identify nonverbal communication
5. Recognize communication barriers
6. Identify techniques for overcoming communication barriers
7. Recognize the elements of oral communication using a sender-receiver process
8. Identify resources and adaptations that are required based on individual needs, i.e., culture and environment, developmental life stage, language, and physical threats to communication
9. Discuss the role of cultural, social, and ethnic diversity in ethical performance of medical assisting practice
10. Discuss the role of assertiveness in effective professional communication
11. Explain how various components of communication can affect the meaning of verbal messages
12. Define active listening
13. List and describe the six interviewing techniques
14. Give an example of how cultural differences may affect communication
15. Discuss how to handle communication problems caused by language barriers
16. List two methods that you can use to promote communication among hearing-, sight-, and speech-impaired patients
17. Discuss how to handle an angry or distressed patient
18. List five actions that you can take to improve communication with a child
19. Discuss your role in communicating with a grieving patient or family member
20. List the five stages of grief as outlined by Elisabeth Kübler-Ross
21. Discuss the key elements of interdisciplinary communication
22. Explore issue of confidentiality as it applies to the medical assistant

Psychomotor Domain

1. Respond to nonverbal communication
2. Use reflection, restatement and clarification techniques to obtain a patient history

Affective Domain

1. Apply active listening skills
2. Use appropriate body language and other nonverbal skills in communicating with patients, family, and staff
3. Demonstrate awareness of the territorial boundaries of the person with whom you are communicating
4. Demonstrate sensitivity appropriate to the message being delivered
5. Demonstrate awareness of how an individual's personal appearance affects anticipated responses
6. Demonstrate recognition of the patient's level of understanding in communications
7. Analyze communication in providing appropriate responses/feedback
8. Recognize and protect personal boundaries in communicating with others
9. Demonstrate respect for individual diversity, incorporating awareness of one's own biases in areas including gender, race, religion, and economic standing
10. Demonstrate empathy in communicating with patients, family, and staff

11. Demonstrate sensitivity in communicating with both providers and patients
12. Respond to issues of confidentiality

ABHES Competencies

1. Identify and respond appropriately when working with/caring for patients with special needs
2. Use empathy when treating terminally ill patients
3. Identify common stages that terminally ill patients go through and list organizations/support groups that can assist patients and family members of patients struggling with terminal illness
4. Advocate on behalf of family/patients, having the ability to deal and communicate with family
5. Analyze the effect of hereditary, cultural, and environmental influences
6. Locate resources and information for patients and employers
7. Be attentive, listen, and learn
8. Be impartial and show empathy when dealing with patients
9. Communicate on the recipient's level of comprehension
10. Serve as liaison between physician and others
11. Recognize and respond to verbal and nonverbal communication

Name: ______________________ Date: ____________ Grade: ____________

COG MULTIPLE CHOICE

Circle the letter preceding the correct answer.

1. Laughing, sobbing, and sighing are examples of:
   a. kinesics.
   b. proxemics.
   c. nonlanguage.
   d. paralanguage.
   e. clarification.

2. Hearing impairment that involves problems with either nerves or the cochlea is called:
   a. anacusis.
   b. conductive.
   c. presbyacusis.
   d. sensorineural.
   e. dysphasia.

3. Sally needs to obtain information from her patient about the medications he is taking. Which of the following open-ended questions is phrased in a way that will elicit the information that Sally needs?
   a. Are you taking your medications?
   b. What medications are you taking?
   c. Have you taken any medications?
   d. Did you take your medications today?
   e. Have you taken medications in the past?

4. Which of the following shows the proper sequence of the sender-receiver process?
   a. Person to send message, message to be sent, person to receive message
   b. Message to be received, person to send message, message to be sent
   c. Message to be sent, person to receive message, person to send message
   d. Person to receive message, person to send message, message to be sent
   e. Person to send message, person to receive message, message to be sent

5. "Those people always get head lice." This statement is an example of:
   a. culture.
   b. demeanor.
   c. discrimination.
   d. stereotyping.
   e. prejudice.

6. What can you do as a medical assistant to communicate effectively with a patient when there is a language barrier?
   a. Find an interpreter who can translate for the patient.
   b. Raise your voice so the patient can focus more on what you are saying.
   c. Give the patient the name and address of a physician who speaks the same language.
   d. Assess the patient and give the physician your best opinion about what is bothering the patient.
   e. Suggest that the patient find another physician who is better equipped to communicate with the patient.

7. When dealing with patients who present communication challenges, such as hearing-impaired or sight-impaired patients, it is best to:
   a. talk about the patient directly with a family member to find out what the problem is.
   b. conduct the interview alone with the patient because he needs to be able to take care of himself.
   c. address the patient's questions in the waiting room, where other people can try to help the patient communicate.
   d. refer the patient to a practice that specializes in working with hearing- and sight-impaired patients.
   e. make sure the patient feels like he is part of the process, even if his condition requires a family member's help.

8. A hearing-impaired patient's test results are in. It is important that the patient gets the results quickly. How should you get the results to the patient?

   a. Mail the test results via priority mail.
   b. Call the patient on a TDD/TTY phone and type in the results.
   c. Drive to the patient's house at lunchtime to deliver the results.
   d. Call an emergency contact of the patient and ask him or her to have the patient make an appointment.
   e. Send the patient a fax containing the test results.

9. Which of the following statements about grieving is true?

   a. The grieving period is approximately 30 days.
   b. Different cultures and individuals demonstrate grief in different ways.
   c. The best way to grieve is through wailing because it lets the emotion out.
   d. The five stages of grief must be followed in that specific order for healing to begin.
   e. Everyone grieves in his or her own way, but all of us go through the stages at the same time.

10. *Proxemics* refers to the:

   a. pitch of a person's voice.
   b. facial expressions a person makes.
   c. physical proximity that people tolerate.
   d. the combination of verbal and nonverbal communication.
   e. the ability of a patient to comprehend difficult messages.

11. Which of the following situations would result in a breach of patient confidentiality?

   a. Shredding unwanted notes that contain patient information
   b. Discussing a patient's lab results with a coworker in the hospital cafeteria
   c. Keeping the glass window between the waiting room and reception desk closed
   d. Shutting down your computer when you leave every night
   e. Paging the physician on an intercom to let him or her know a patient is waiting on the phone for results

12. "Those results can't be true. The doctor must have mixed me up with another patient." This statement reflects which of the following stages of grieving?

   a. Anger
   b. Denial
   c. Depression
   d. Bargaining
   e. Acceptance

13. Which of the following statements about communication is correct?

   a. Communication can be either verbal or nonverbal.
   b. Written messages can be interpreted through paralanguage.
   c. Verbal communication involves both oral communication and body language.
   d. Body language is the most important form of communication.
   e. Touch should be avoided in all forms of communication because it makes the recipient of the message uncomfortable.

14. During a patient interview, repeating what you have heard the patient say using an open-ended statement is called:

   a. clarifying.
   b. reflecting.
   c. summarizing.
   d. paraphrasing.
   e. allowing silences.

15. What should you do during a patient interview if there is silence?

a. Silence should not be allowed during a patient interview.

b. Immediately start talking so the patient does not feel awkward.

c. Fill in charts that need to be completed until the patient is ready.

d. Wait for the physician to arrive to speak with the patient.

e. Gather your thoughts and think of any additional questions you have.

16. The physician is behind schedule, and a patient is angry that her appointment is late. The best way to deal with the patient is to:

a. tell her anything that will calm her down.

b. ignore her until the problem is solved.

c. threaten that the physician will no longer treat her if she continues to complain.

d. keep her informed of when the physician will be able to see her.

e. ask her why it is such a big deal.

17. Why is it helpful to ask open-ended questions during a patient interview?

a. They let the patient give yes or no answers.

b. They let the patient develop an answer and explain it.

c. They let the patient respond quickly using few words.

d. They provide simple answers that are easy to note in the chart.

e. They let the patient give his or her own feelings and opinions on the subject.

18. Difficulty with speech is called:

a. dysphasia.

b. dysphonia.

c. nyctalopia.

d. strabismus.

e. myopia.

19. One particular physician runs behind schedule most of the time. His CMA has to work until he finishes seeing his patients, but her child must be picked up from day-care by 6:00 p.m. Which statement below represents one of an assertive person?

a. I won't work late another day! My hours are 8:00 a.m. to 5:00 p.m.

b. Sorry, doctor, I'm out of here to pick up my child. Someone else will have to stay.

c. My daughter must be picked up by 6:00 every day. Could we look at the possibility of taking turns staying late? I could make arrangements for one day out of the week.

d. Since you are the reason we run late, you should take care of the patients yourself.

e. I can't believe you're asking me to stay late again. I am going to find another job.

20. The limit of personal space is generally considered to be a:

a. 1-foot radius.

b. 3-foot radius.

c. 5-foot radius.

d. 10-foot radius.

e. 15-foot radius.

COG MATCHING

Grade: ____________

Match the following key terms to their definitions.

Key Terms	Definitions
21. _____ anacusis	**a.** information
22. _____ bias	**b.** something that is beneficial to a patient
23. _____ clarification	**c.** a group of people who share a way of life and beliefs
24. _____ cultures	**d.** holding an opinion of all members of a particular culture, race, religion, or age group based on oversimplified or negative characterizations
25. _____ demeanor	**e.** loss of hearing associated with aging
26. _____ discrimination	**f.** difficulty speaking
27. _____ dysphasia	**g.** sounds that include laughing, sobbing, sighing, or grunting to convey information
28. _____ dysphonia	**h.** the response to a message
29. _____ feedback	**i.** restating what a person said using your own words or phrases
30. _____ grief	**j.** removal of confusion or uncertainty
31. _____ messages	**k.** formation of an opinion without foundation or reason
32. _____ mourning	**l.** a demonstration of the signs of grief
33. _____ nonlanguage	**m.** complete hearing loss
34. _____ paralanguage	**n.** briefly reviewing information discussed to determine the patient's comprehension
35. _____ paraphrasing	**o.** great sadness caused by a loss
36. _____ presbyacusis	**p.** voice tone, quality, volume, pitch, and range
37. _____ reflecting	**q.** the way a person looks, behaves, and conducts himself
38. _____ stereotyping	**r.** a voice impairment that is caused by a physical condition, such as oral surgery
39. _____ summarizing	**s.** the act of not treating a patient fairly or respectfully because of his cultural, social, or personal values
40. _____ therapeutic	**t.** repeating what one heard using open-ended questions

COG IDENTIFICATION

Grade: ___________

41. The two main forms of communication are verbal communication and nonverbal communication. Read each form of communication below and place an "A" for verbal or a "B" for nonverbal in the space provided.

a. _____ A patient sighs while explaining her symptoms.

b. _____ A patient shrugs his shoulders after being told he needs to lose weight.

c. _____ A patient's eyes dart around the room during an explanation of a procedure.

d. _____ A physician writes "take two aspirin every 8 hours."

e. _____ A mother is given a sheet of paper describing what to expect of her baby during months 6–9.

f. _____ A physician puts her hand on a patient's shoulder before delivering test results.

COG PSY SHORT ANSWER

Grade: ___________

42. List five local resources that can assist a grieving patient or family member. Include the name of the agency, type of help that it offers, and its phone number.

____

____

____

43. Why is it important to respect cultural diversity?

____

____

____

44. List the five stages of grief as outlined by Elisabeth Kübler-Ross.

____

____

____

45. List five actions that you can take to improve communication with a child.

46. List two methods that you can use to promote communication among hearing-, sight-, and speech-impaired patients.

47. List and describe the six interviewing techniques.

48. List two major forms of communication.

49. What is the difference between aggressiveness and assertiveness?

AFF WHAT WOULD YOU DO?

Grade: ____________

50. You are working in the reception area of a busy medical practice. Patients come and go all day long, and it is your responsibility to move the flow along. One particularly busy day, you are registering an 89-year-old man. You ask him to read and sign an authorization to release records to Medicare. He says that he cannot see the form and asks if his wife can sign. His nonverbal cues make you wonder if he can read and write. From the list below, choose all appropriate actions.

a. Ask him if he would like the number for an adult literacy program.

b. Tell him that his wife can sign for him, but she should also read the authorization for him.

c. Have his wife initial the "signature" and then you sign as a witness.

d. Tell him to make an "X" if he cannot write.

e. Tell him to sign the form without reading it.

51. A patient calls the office with symptoms and a condition that you are not familiar with. She has used some terms that you do not understand. When you relay the message to the physician, how should you communicate the patient's problem?

____

____

____

COG AFF IDENTIFICATION

Grade: ____________

52. Read the list of nonverbal communication cues below. Beside each one, list the problem or issue this action might indicate:

a. Crossed arms ____________________

b. Slumping in chair ____________________

c. A child hiding behind mother ____________________

d. Hand clenching ____________________

53. Physicians use the information obtained during a patient interview to help them assess the patient's health. Patients will be more willing to provide information during a professionally conducted interview. Read each of the following statements describing patient interviews. Answer "yes" if the statement describes a correct interview practice; answer "no" if it describes an incorrect interview practice. Provide an explanation on how to correct the problem for all no answers.

a. Patient interviews can be conducted in an exam room or in the waiting room. ________________

b. Answering a phone call in the middle of a new patient interview is acceptable if it is a call you have been waiting for. ________________

c. It is important to maintain eye contact with the patient, so you do not write any patient responses down until the interview is over. ________________

d. You confirm which blood pressure medication and what dosage the patient is taking. ________________

e. There is nothing wrong with skipping questions in a patient interview that may make the patient feel uncomfortable. ________________

f. Introducing yourself to the patient is a nice way to start an interview. ________________

COG TRUE OR FALSE?

Grade: ________

Determine whether the following statements are true or false. If false, explain why.

54. When the office is busy, it is okay to refer to patients by their medical conditions, for example, "stomach pain in room 1."

____

55. If an older adult patient does not have a ride home, a staff member in the office should offer him or her one.

____

56. When talking with patients, do not reveal too many personal details about your life.

____

57. It is inappropriate to carry on personal conversations with other staff members in front of a patient.

____

PSY ACTIVE LEARNING

Grade: ____________

58. Practice active listening with a partner. Have your partner tell you a detailed story that you have never heard before or explain a topic that you are unfamiliar with. After he or she has finished, wait silently for 2 minutes. Then, try to repeat the story or steps back to your partner. Next, reverse roles and let your partner listen while you tell a story or explain a concept.

____

____

____

59. If you work in a pediatric office, you will certainly spend a good deal of time communicating with children. To help strengthen your communication skills with children, find a local preschool or elementary school teacher who has experience working with children. Interview this teacher about his or her communication techniques and write a list of 10 tips for communicating with children.

____

____

____

AFF CASE STUDY FOR CRITICAL THINKING A

Grade: ____________

You are working in a geriatric office taking patients back, and one of your patients is a Spanish-speaking woman who comes into the office with her son and daughter. Her body language indicates fear and worry. She appears very shy and depends on her son and daughter for assistance. They speak a little bit of English, but it is difficult to communicate with them.

60. Your first duty is to interview the patient about her medical history. Of the following steps, circle the ones you should take to get information.

a. Speak in a normal tone and volume.

b. Speak directly to the son and daughter.

c. When asking a question about eyesight, point to your eyes.

d. Use abbreviations and slang terms for medical tests.

e. Ask the woman's son to be the interpreter and her daughter to wait outside.

f. Use complex medical language to explain procedures.

g. Use a Spanish-to-English dictionary.

61. The physician will be doing a complete exam on the patient. She must change into a gown. You have everyone but her daughter leave the exam room. You hand a gown to her daughter who starts toward her mother to help the patient change. The patient backs up into the corner of the room. Of the following actions, which ONE is the most appropriate?

a. Take the gown from the daughter and give it to the patient.

b. Leave the room and let the daughter handle it.

c. Tell her that she will be covered and you have a blanket for her if she is cold.

d. Tell the physician that the patient would not undress and let him or her handle it.

e. Give the patient a big hug—that should make her feel better.

62. Following a difficult exam, the physician notes a suspicious mole on the patient's back. He instructs you to get her an appointment with a dermatologist. You explain to the three of them that you will make an appointment. You ask them if they have a preference, and they appear confused. Circle all appropriate actions in the list below.

a. Give them a patient brochure on moles.

b. Make an appointment in 2 weeks for them to return with a translator.

c. Make the appointment, and write down the name and address of the facility.

d. Give the patient a big hug and tell her what a brave girl she was.

e. Use a Spanish-to-English dictionary to try to explain.

AFF CASE STUDY FOR CRITICAL THINKING B

Grade: ____________

63. Your physician is treating a 7-year-old girl who needs to have her tonsils removed. Her mother has 60% hearing loss and depends on lip-reading to communicate. You need to have her sign paperwork and explain the child's need for a pre-anesthesia appointment at the hospital. Circle the suggestions below that will help you to communicate with her.

a. Gently touch the patient to get her attention.

b. Exaggerate your facial movements.

c. Eliminate all distractions.

d. Enunciate clearly.

e. Use short sentences with short words.

f. Speak loudly.

g. Give the patient written instructions.

h. Turn toward the light so your face is illuminated.

i. Talk face-to-face with the patient, not at an angle.

64. Protocol dictates that the child has a history and physical exam before her surgery. She is obviously afraid and confused about what is happening. Circle the actions listed below that would be appropriate when communicating with the child.

a. Tell the child when you need to touch him or her and what you are going to do.

b. Talk loudly and sternly so the child will stay focused on you and not other distractions in the office.

c. Work quickly and let him or her be surprised by what you do.

d. Rephrase questions until the child understands.

e. Be playful to help gain the child's cooperation.

f. Try to speak to children at their eye level.

CHAPTER 4

Patient Education

Learning Outcomes

Cognitive Domain

1. Spell and define the key terms
2. Explain the medical assistant's role in patient education
3. Define the five steps in the patient education process
4. Identify five conditions that are needed for patient education to occur
5. Explain Maslow's hierarchy of human needs
6. List five factors that may hinder patient education and at least two methods to compensate for each of these factors
7. Discuss five preventive medicine guidelines that you should teach your patients
8. Explain the kinds of information that should be included in patient teaching about medication therapy
9. Explain your role in teaching patients about alternative medicine therapies
10. List and explain relaxation techniques that you and patients can learn to help with stress management
11. Describe how to prepare a teaching plan
12. List potential sources of patient education materials
13. Locate community resources and list ways of organizing and disseminating information
14. Recognize communication barriers
15. Identify techniques for overcoming communication barriers
16. Identify resources and adaptations that are required based on individual needs i.e. cuture and environment, developmental life stage, language, and physical threats to communication

Psychomotor Domain

1. Document patient education (Procedure 4-1)
2. Develop and maintain a current list of community resources related to the patient's health care needs (Procedure 4-2)

Affective Domain

1. Use language/verbal skills that enable patients' understanding
2. Demonstrate respect for diversity in approaching patients and families
3. Demonstrate empathy in communicating with patients, family and staff
4. Demonstrate sensitivity appropriate to the message being delivered
5. Demonstrate recognition of the patient's level of understanding in communications
6. Demonstrate sensitivity to patient rights

ABHES Competencies

1. Identify and respond appropriately when working/caring for patients with special needs
2. Adapt to individualized needs
3. Communicate on the recipient's level of comprehension
4. Be impartial and show empathy when dealing with patients

Name: ______________________________ Date: ______________ Grade: ______________

COG MULTIPLE CHOICE

Circle the BEST answer.

1. During assessment, the most comprehensive source from which to obtain patient information is the:
   a. physician's notes.
   b. immunization record.
   c. medical record.
   d. family member.
   e. nurse.

2. When teaching a patient with many chronic health problems, it is important to
   a. focus on each problem separately.
   b. tell them that your grandmother has many of the same problems.
   c. bond with him or her.
   d. have the patient come back another time with a family member.
   e. have the physician talk to him or her.

3. Which of the following is an example of a psychomotor skill that a patient may perform?
   a. Telling the physician about his or her symptoms
   b. Explaining how a part of the body is feeling
   c. Walking around with a crutch
   d. Watching television in the waiting room
   e. Listening to a physician's instructions

4. Which part of Maslow's pyramid is the point at which a patient has satisfied all basic needs and feels he or she has control over his or her life?
   a. Safety and security
   b. Esteem
   c. Self-actualization
   d. Affection
   e. Physiologic

5. Noncompliance occurs when the patient:
   a. experiences a decrease in symptoms healed.
   b. forgets to pay his or her bill.
   c. refuses to follow the physician's orders.
   d. requests a new medical assistant to assist the physician.
   e. agrees with the physician.

6. The power of believing that something will make you better when there is no chemical reaction that warrants such improvement is:
   a. self-relaxation.
   b. positive stress.
   c. acupuncture.
   d. placebo.
   e. visualization.

7. Patient education should consist of multiple techniques or approaches so:
   a. the patient can apply his or her new knowledge to real-life events.
   b. the patient will learn and retain more.
   c. the patient will understand that there are many ways to look at an issue.
   d. the patient will know where you stand on his or her health care options.
   e. the patient will have a wider choice of treatments.

8. One mental health illness that can hinder patient education is:
   a. diabetes.
   b. Lyme disease.
   c. obstructive pulmonary disease.
   d. Alzheimer disease.
   e. anemia.

9. Health assessment forms that assess a patient's education level may also help you determine a patient's ability to:

a. read.

b. listen.

c. communicate.

d. respond.

e. evaluate.

10. Before developing a medication schedule, you should evaluate the patient's:

a. prescribed medication.

b. side effects.

c. changes in bodily functions.

d. daily routine.

e. bowel movements.

11. Which is an example of a recommended preventive procedure?

a. Regular teeth whitening

b. Childhood immunizations

c. Daily exercise

d. Yearly lung cancer evaluations

e. Occasional antibiotics

12. Which of the following is true of herbal supplements?

a. A medical assistant can recommend that a patient start taking herbal supplements without the physician's approval.

b. A health store clerk is a good source of information on supplements.

c. Products that claim to detoxify the whole body are generally effective.

d. Supplements will not interfere with blood sugar levels because they are not medication.

e. Patients should be advised that because a product is natural does not mean it is safe.

13. One example of a physiologic response to negative stress is:

a. elevated mood.

b. hunger pangs.

c. headache.

d. profuse bleeding.

e. energy boost.

14. In Maslow's hierarchy of needs, air, water, food, and rest are considered:

a. affection needs.

b. safety and security needs.

c. esteem needs.

d. self-actualization needs.

e. physiologic needs.

15. When explaining the benefits and risks of a proposed treatment to a patient who uses American Sign Language to communicate, the physician must:

a. be sure the patient is given the information in writing.

b. provide a sign language interpreter if the patient does not bring one.

c. make the patient feel comfortable.

d. use a notepad to communicate.

e. let the medical assistant handle it.

16. Humans use defense mechanisms to:

a. cope with painful problems.

b. increase their sense of accomplishment.

c. decrease effects of chronic physical pain.

d. learn to get along well with others.

e. explain complicated emotions to medical staff.

17. Support groups give patients the opportunity to:

a. exchange and compare medical records.

b. meet and share ideas with others who are experiencing the same issues.

c. spread the good word about the medical office.

d. obtain their basic physiologic needs.

e. learn more about malpractice suits.

18. When selecting teaching material, you should first:

a. choose preprinted material.

b. create your own material.

c. assess your patient's general level of understanding.

d. let the patient find a book from the clinic library.

e. ask the patient to create a list of specific questions.

19. Acupressure is different from acupuncture because:

a. it does not use needles.

b. it is not an alternative medicine.

c. it cannot be used with cancer patients.

d. it does not require any licensure.

e. it is less effective.

20. If your community does not have a central agency for information and resources, then you should create a(n):

a. hierarchy of needs.

b. teaching plan.

c. telephone directory.

d. information sheet.

e. flowchart.

21. Suppose you want to teach a patient about the need to adopt a low-sugar diet because of diabetes, but the patient doesn't believe that diabetes is a serious health problem. If education is to be effective, then which of the following must the patient accept? Circle all that apply.

a. Diabetes has to be managed.

b. There is a correlation between high sugar intake and diabetes.

c. Diabetes isn't as serious as other diseases.

d. Diabetes management requires dietary changes.

e. It is possible to consume large quantities of high-sugar foods, but only occasionally.

COG MATCHING

Grade: ________

Match the following key terms to their definitions.

Key Terms

22. _____ alternative treatment
23. _____ assessment
24. _____ coping mechanisms
25. _____ dissemination
26. _____ documentation
27. _____ evaluation
28. _____ implementation
29. _____ learning objectives
30. _____ noncompliance
31. _____ placebo effect
32. _____ planning

Definitions

a. involves using the information you have gathered to determine how you will approach the patient's learning needs

b. skill that requires the patient to physically perform a task

c. the process that indicates how well patients are adapting or applying new information to their lives

d. produced by illness or injury and may result in physiological and psychological effects

e. includes procedures or tasks that will be discussed or performed at various points in the program to help achieve the goal

f. the process of distributing information on community resources

g. includes recording of all teachings that occurred

h. the patient's inability or refusal to follow a prescribed order

i. involves gathering information about the patient's present health care needs and abilities

33. _____ psychomotor

34. _____ stress

j. psychological defenses employed to help deal with the painful and difficult problems life can bring

k. the power of believing that something will make you better when there is no chemical reaction that warrants such improvement

l. the expected outcomes for the teaching process

m. an option or substitute to the standard medical treatment such as acupuncture

SHORT ANSWER

Grade: _______

35. List three potential sources of patient education materials.

____

____

____

36. List and explain three relaxation techniques that you and patients can learn to help with stress management.

____

____

____

AFF WHAT WOULD YOU DO?

Grade: _______

37. You work in a pediatric practice. A mother brings her 6-month-old son in for a routine checkup. The child has a visible lump on the right side of his head, just above his ear. The mother states that the child fell off a twin bed when she was changing his diaper. After examining the child, the physician asks you to instruct the mother in safety and also have her watch the baby closely for the next few days for signs of concussion.

A. What resources might be available to you?

____

____

B. How might you evaluate the mother's barriers to communication and understanding?

____

____

C. What method of instruction would you use for this situation?

____

____

D. What would your teaching plan need to include?

____

____

E. What measures should be taken if the child's injuries were consistent with possible abuse?

____

____

F. Why is patient education important?

____

____

38. Write a sentence explaining why, as a medical assistant, you must set aside your own personal feelings and life experiences when educating patients.

____

____

____

COG IDENTIFICATION

Grade: ________

List the five factors that can hinder patient education.

39. ______________________________

40. ______________________________

41. ______________________________

42. ______________________________

43. ______________________________

COG PSY ACTIVE LEARNING

Grade: _______

44. Juggling school with other commitments may occasionally cause negative stress in your life. Make a list of how you experience stress in your daily life. Then, choose one of the three relaxation techniques discussed in this chapter. Practice that technique and then write a paragraph describing the "pros" and "cons" of the chosen technique.

____

____

____

45. Develop a teaching plan for a family member or friend. For example, if your mother has asthma, then do research on the Internet to find information and resources about asthma. Remember to include all of the elements of a teaching plan. Practice your teaching techniques by educating a family member or friend about a particular illness or disease.

____

____

____

46. Choose a health concern that may require external support. For example, a patient fighting cancer may wish to join a support group or other organization for help. Search the Internet for local, state, and national agencies that provide information, support, and services to patients with your chosen need. Then, compile this information in an informative and creative brochure, pamphlet, or other learning tool.

____

____

____

COG PSY PATIENT EDUCATION

Grade: _______

47. A patient wants to use alternative medicine in addition to medicine prescribed by the physician. What should you do?

____

____

____

48. A patient in your care is suffering physiologic effects from negative stress brought on by chronic back pain. What types of coping strategies would you recommend to the patient and why?

____

____

____

49. Julia is an 8-year-old patient who has been diagnosed with type 1 diabetes. The medical office has a preprinted teaching plan entitled "Living with Type 2 Diabetes." Should you use this plan or develop your own? Explain.

____

____

____

TRUE OR FALSE?

Grade: ________

Determine whether the following statements are true or false. If false, explain why.

50. Patients benefit from the use of teaching aids that they can take home and use as reference material.

____

51. If a patient asks you a question and you're not sure of the answer, then you should give your best guess.

____

52. A patient must have his basic needs met before self-actualization may occur.

____

53. Visualization is a relaxation technique that involves deep-breathing and physical exercise.

____

AFF CASE STUDY FOR CRITICAL THINKING A

Grade: ________

A 5-year-old girl in your pediatric practice has just been diagnosed with juvenile diabetes. Your physician asks you to assist the patient's parents with resources available to them.

54. From the following list, circle the BEST resource.

- **a.** Materials from a pharmaceutical company
- **b.** Other patients who have this problem
- **c.** The official website of the American Diabetes Association
- **d.** Another pediatrician's office
- **e.** American Medical Technologists, Inc.

55. When developing a teaching plan, circle the most appropriate entry under Learning Objectives?

- **a.** Patient not involved in training due to age
- **b.** Patient's mother describes the body's use of insulin
- **c.** See documentation of patient education in chart
- **d.** Gave patient instructional video: "Your Child and Diabetes"
- **e.** Patient understands disease

AFF CASE STUDY FOR CRITICAL THINKING B

Grade: ________

Your physician instructs you to come up with a plan for Mr. Johns who has been diagnosed with hypercholesterolemia. He needs to change his eating habits and lifestyle drastically. You plan to help him form a plan for making these changes.

56. Patients should be encouraged to take an active approach to their health and health care education. To assist Mr. Johns effectively, which of the following must you do? Circle all that apply.

- **a.** Help Mr. Johns accept his illness.
- **b.** Expect Mr. Johns to follow your instructions without further explanation.
- **c.** Involve Mr. Johns in the process of gaining knowledge.
- **d.** Provide Mr. Johns with positive reinforcement.
- **e.** Give Mr. Johns the most in-depth professional textbooks you can find.

57. Your plan for Mr. Johns should include all of the following EXCEPT:

a. A timeline for a gradually progressing walking program
b. recipes for low-fat dishes
c. pamphlets with information about his condition
d. documentation of your instruction
e. a list of his medications

58. Ms. Jasinski is an older adult patient who has recently lost several relatives and friends. She lives alone, feels disconnected from others and, as a result, her health has begun to deteriorate. Brian, a medical assistant, gives Ms. Jasinski a friendly hug when he sees her during patient visits. He talks to her and listens to her stories. He has also encouraged her to join a senior citizens' group. Circle which of Maslow's hierarchy of needs has Brian helped fulfill for Ms. Jasinski?

a. physiological
b. safety and security
c. affection and belonging
d. self-actualization

PSY PROCEDURE 4-1 Document Patient Education

Name: ______________________ Date: ________ Time: ________ Grade: ________

EQUIPMENT/SUPPLIES: Patient's chart, pen

STANDARDS: Given the needed equipment and a place to work, the student will perform this skill with ______% accuracy in a total of ______ minutes. *(Your instructor will tell you what the percentage and time limits will be before you begin.)*

KEY: 4 = Satisfactory 0 = Unsatisfactory NA = This step is not counted

PROCEDURE STEPS	SELF	PARTNER	INSTRUCTOR
1. Record the date and time of teaching.	☐	☐	☐
2. Record the information taught.	☐	☐	☐
3. Record the manner in which the information was taught.	☐	☐	☐
4. Record your evaluation of your teaching.	☐	☐	☐
5. Record any additional teaching planned.	☐	☐	☐
6. AFF Explain what you would do if you forgot to document an action you took during the patient education process.	☐	☐	☐

____

____

____

____

Note: The medical assistant may sign his or her name in the patient record using only the "CMA" credential if the office has a signature log denoting the entire credential as "CMA(AAMA)."

CALCULATION

Total Possible Points: ______

Total Points Earned: ______ Multiplied by 100 = ______ Divided by Total Possible Points = ______ %

PASS ☐ **FAIL** ☐ **COMMENTS:**

Student's signature ______________________ Date ______

Partner's signature ______________________ Date ______

Instructor's signature ______________________ Date ______

PSY PROCEDURE 4-2 Develop and Maintain a Current List of Community Resources Related to Patients' Healthcare Needs

Name: ______________________ Date: __________ Time: __________ Grade: __________

EQUIPMENT/SUPPLIES: Phone book, Internet, newspaper

STANDARDS: Given the needed equipment and a place to work, the student will perform this skill with ______% accuracy in a total of ______ minutes. *(Your instructor will tell you what the percentage and time limits will be before you begin.)*

KEY: 4 = Satisfactory 0 = Unsatisfactory NA = This step is not counted

PROCEDURE STEPS	SELF	PARTNER	INSTRUCTOR
1. Assess the patient's needs for the following: **a.** Education **b.** Someone to talk to **c.** Financial information **d.** Support groups **e.** Home health needs	☐	☐	☐
2. Check the local telephone book for local and state resources.	☐	☐	☐
3. Check for Web sites for the city and/or county in which the patient lives.	☐	☐	☐
4. Be prepared with materials already on hand.	☐	☐	☐
5. Give the patient the contact information in writing.	☐	☐	☐
6. Document actions and the information given to the patient.	☐	☐	☐
7. Instruct the patient to contact the office if he has any difficulty.	☐	☐	☐
8. AFF Explain what suggestions or assistance you would offer to a patient who would benefit from online patient education resources but does not own a computer.	☐	☐	☐

___

___

___

CALCULATION

Total Possible Points: ______

Total Points Earned: ______ Multiplied by 100 = ______ Divided by Total Possible Points = ______ %

PASS **FAIL** **COMMENTS:**

☐ ☐

Student's signature ________________________________ Date ______

Partner's signature ________________________________ Date ______

Instructor's signature ________________________________ Date ______

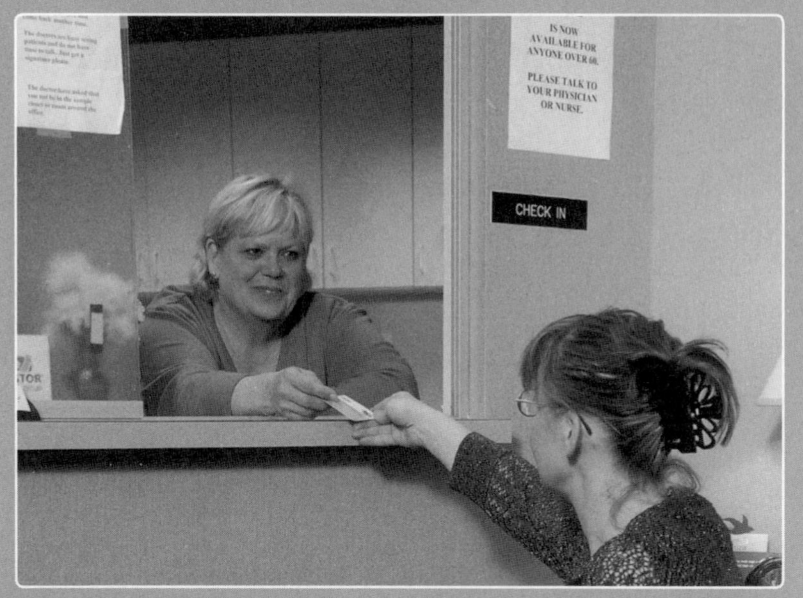

PART

II

The Administrative Medical Assistant

UNIT TWO

Fundamentals of Administrative Medical Assisting

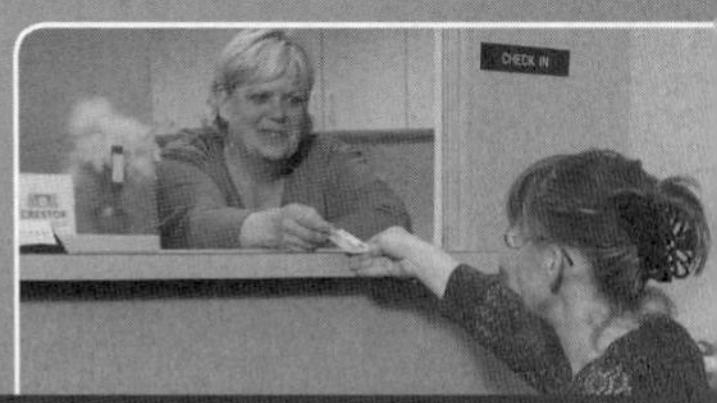

CHAPTER 5

The First Contact: Telephone and Reception

Learning Outcomes

Cognitive Domain

1. Spell and define the key terms
2. Explain the importance of displaying a professional image to all patients
3. List six duties of the medical office receptionist
4. List four sources from which messages can be retrieved
5. Discuss various steps that can be taken to promote good ergonomics
6. Describe the basic guidelines for waiting room environments
7. Describe the proper method for maintaining infection control standards in the waiting room
8. Discuss the five basic guidelines for telephone use
9. Describe the types of incoming telephone calls received by the medical office
10. Discuss how to identify and handle callers with medical emergencies
11. Describe how to triage incoming calls
12. List the information that should be given to an emergency medical service dispatcher
13. Describe the types of telephone services and special features
14. Discuss applications of electronic technology in effective communication

Psychomotor Domain

1. Handle incoming calls (Procedure 5-1)
   - Demonstrate telephone techniques
2. Call Emergency Medical Services (Procedure 5-2)
   - Demonstrate self awareness in responding to emergency situations
   - Recognize the effects of stress on all persons involved in emergency situations
3. Explain general office policies (Procedure 5-3)
   - Report relevant information to others succinctly and accurately
4. Verify eligibility for managed care services

Affective Domain

1. Demonstrate empathy in communicating with patients, family, and staff
2. Implement time management principles to maintain effective office function
3. Communicate in language the patient can understand regarding managed care and insurance plans
4. Demonstrate awareness of the consequences of not working within the legal scope of practice
5. Demonstrate sensitivity in communicating with both providers and patients
6. Demonstrate sensitivity to patient rights

ABHES Competencies

1. Use proper telephone technique
2. Receive, organize, prioritize, and transmit information expediently
3. Apply electronic technology

Name: ______________________ Date: __________ Grade: __________

COG MULTIPLE CHOICE

1. Which of the following creates a professional image?
   - a. Arguing with a patient
   - b. Clean, pressed clothing
   - c. Brightly colored fingernails
   - d. Referring to the physicians by his or her first name
   - e. Expensive flowery perfume

2. How can you exercise diplomacy?
   - a. Treat patients as they treat you.
   - b. Treat patients as you would like to be treated.
   - c. Ignore patients who complain about their illnesses.
   - d. Answer patients' questions about other patients they see in the waiting room.
   - e. Disclose confidential information if a patient or relative asks for it tactfully.

3. When preparing the charts for the day, the charts should be put in order by:
   - a. age.
   - b. last name.
   - c. chart number.
   - d. reason for visit.
   - e. appointment time.

4. The receptionist should check phone messages:
   - a. at night before leaving.
   - b. in the morning when coming in.
   - c. when on the phone and knowing a call has gone to voice mail.
   - d. only after breaks, because each call coming in should be answered.
   - e. when the office opens, after breaks, and periodically throughout the day.

5. Triaging calls is important because:
   - a. it reduces the amount of time that callers wait.
   - b. it places the calls in order of most urgent to least urgent.
   - c. it lets the receptionist take care of the calls as quickly as possible.
   - d. it puts the calls in time order so the receptionist knows who called first.
   - e. it makes it easier for the receptionist to see which calls will be the easiest to handle.

6. There is a sign in the pediatrician's office that says "Do not throw dirty diapers in the garbage." Which of the following choices best explains the reason for the sign?
   - a. Dirty diapers cannot be recycled.
   - b. Dirty diapers are biohazardous waste.
   - c. Dirty diapers could leave an offensive odor.
   - d. Dirty diapers could make the garbage too heavy.
   - e. Dirty diapers take up too much room in the garbage.

7. Chewing gum or eating while on the phone could interfere with a person's:
   - a. diction.
   - b. attitude.
   - c. ergonomics.
   - d. expression.
   - e. pronunciation.

8. Which of the following activities should a receptionist do in the morning to prepare the office for patients?
   - a. Vacuum the office.
   - b. Stock office supplies.
   - c. Disinfect examination rooms.
   - d. Turn on printers and copiers.
   - e. Clean the patient restrooms.

9. Which of the following statements about telephone courtesy is correct?

a. If two lines are ringing at once, answer one call and let the other go to voice mail.

b. If you are on the other line, it is acceptable to let the phone ring until you can answer it.

c. If a caller is upset, leaving him or her on hold will help improve the caller's attitude.

d. If you need to answer another line, ask if the caller would mind holding and wait for a response.

e. If someone is on hold for more than 90 seconds, he or she must leave a message and someone will call them back.

10. An ergonomic workstation is beneficial because it:

a. prevents injuries to employees.

b. educates patients about disease.

c. maintains patients' confidentiality.

d. creates a soothing, relaxed atmosphere.

e. prevents the spread of contagious diseases.

11. Which feature fosters a positive waiting room environment?

a. Abstract artwork on the walls

b. Only sofas for patients to sit in

c. Soap operas on the waiting room television

d. Prominent display of the office fax machine

e. Patient education materials in the reception area

12. When a patient calls the office and wants to be seen for chest pain, your first action should be

a. Ask if he or she also has shortness of breath, nausea, and/or profuse sweating.

b. Tell him or her to hang up and call 911.

c. Asks the patient's name in case he or she loses consciousness.

d. Tell the patient to make sure his front door is unlocked.

e. Give the patient an appointment for the next day.

13. A 5-year-old girl has just come into the office with her mother. She has the flu and is vomiting into a plastic bag. Which of the following should the receptionist do?

a. Get the patient into an examination room.

b. Call the hospital and request an ambulance.

c. Tell her to sit near the bathroom so she can vomit in the toilet.

d. Place a new plastic bag in your garbage can and ask the girl to use it.

e. Ask the patient to wait outside and you will get her when it is her turn.

14. An angry patient calls the office demanding to speak to the physician. The physician is not in the office. What should the receptionist do?

a. Page the physician immediately.

b. Try to calm the patient and take a message.

c. Give the caller the physician's cell phone number.

d. Tell the patient to calm down and call back in an hour.

e. Place the patient on hold until he or she has calmed down.

15. Which of the following statements about e-mail is true?

a. Patient e-mails should be deleted from the computer.

b. The receptionist does not generally have access to e-mail.

c. Actions taken in regard to e-mail do not need to be documented.

d. Patients should not e-mail the office under any circumstances.

e. E-mails should not be printed because the wrong person could view them.

16. The best technique for preventing the spread of disease is:

a. washing your hands after any contact with patients.

b. placing very sick patients immediately in an exam room.

c. removing all reading materials or toys from the waiting room.

d. keeping the window to the reception area closed at all times.

e. preventing patients from changing channels on the TV in the waiting room.

17. One way to ensure patient privacy in the reception area is to:

a. take all the patient's information at the front desk.

b. ask the patient's permission before placing her name on the sign-in sheet.

c. use computers in examination rooms only.

d. make telephone calls regarding referrals at the front desk.

e. close the privacy window when you are not speaking with a patient.

18. When receiving a call from a lab regarding a patient's test results, you should post the information:

a. as an e-mail to the physician.

b. in the receptionist's notebook.

c. in the front of the patient's chart.

d. as an e-mail to the patient's insurance company.

e. in the front of the physician's appointment book.

19. In case of an emergency in the physician's office, who is usually responsible for calling emergency medical services (EMS)?

a. Physician

b. Dispatcher

c. Receptionist

d. Clinical staff

e. Patient's relatives

20. When calling EMS for a patient who has an abnormal EKG, which of the following should be given first?

a. The patient's name and age

b. Your location

c. The patient's insurance carrier

d. The patient's problem

e. Where they will be taking the patient

COG MATCHING

Grade: ______

Match the following key terms to their definitions.

Key Terms

21. ____ attitude

22. ____ closed captioning

23. ____ diction

24. ____ diplomacy

25. ____ emergency medical service (EMS)

26. ____ ergonomic

27. ____ receptionist

28. ____ teletypewriter (TTY)

29. ____ triage

Definitions

a. a person who performs administrative tasks and greets patients as they arrive at an office

b. the art of handling people with tact and genuine concern

c. a group of health care workers who care for sick and injured patients on the way to a hospital

d. printed words displayed on a television screen to help people with hearing disabilities or impairments

e. describing a workstation designed to prevent work-related injuries

f. the style of speaking and enunciating words

g. the sorting of patients into categories based on their level of sickness or injury

h. a state of mind or feeling regarding some matter

i. a special machine that allows communication on a telephone with a hearing-impaired person

COG SHORT ANSWER

Grade: ______

30. List the four sources of messages to be collected by the receptionist.

______

______

______

______

31. Why is it important to keep the waiting area neat and clean?

______

______

______

______

32. List the types of incoming calls received by the medical office.

____

____

____

____

33. Infection control is important to prevent the spread of disease among patients. List three things a medical assistant can do to help with infection control.

____

____

____

____

34. List four things you can do to maintain patient confidentiality within the reception area and waiting room.

____

____

____

____

35. You are training a new receptionist. She doesn't understand why triaging calls is important. How would you explain this to her?

____

____

____

____

PSY IDENTIFICATION

Grade: ____________

36. The waiting room should be a comfortable and safe place for patients to wait. Review the list of guidelines below and determine which contribute to a comfortable and safe waiting room environment. Place a check in the "Yes" column for those guidelines that contribute to a comfortable and safe waiting room and place a check in the "No" column for those that do not.

Task	Yes	No
a. Sofas are preferable because they fit more people.		
b. Provide only chairs without arms.		
c. Bright, primary colors are more suitable and cheery.		
d. The room should be well ventilated and kept at a comfortable temperature.		
e. Soothing background music is acceptable.		
f. Reading material, like current magazines, should be provided.		
g. Patients should be allowed to control the television.		
h. In an office for adults, anything can be watched on the television.		
i. Closed captioning should be offered to patients with hearing impairments who want to watch television.		

37. A patient comes into the office with a severe bloody nose. He leaves bloody tissues in the waiting room and got blood on a magazine and a chair. Your supervisor says to you, "Come on! Get some gloves. We've got to clean this right away." Why do you need gloves? Why is it important that the waiting room be cleaned immediately?

____

____

____

____

COG TRUE OR FALSE?

Grade: ____________

As a receptionist, you'll be answering incoming calls. Review the statements below and place a check in the "True" column for those that are true and place a check in the "False" column for those that are false.

Incoming Calls	True	False
38. Always ask new patients for their phone number in case you need to call them back.		
39. Always give patients an exact quote for services if asked.		
40. Patient information cannot be given to anyone without the patient's consent.		
41. All laboratory results phoned into the office must be immediately brought to the physician's attention.		
42. When a nursing home calls with a satisfactory report about a patient, you should take the information down, record it in the patient's chart, and place it on the physician's desk for review.		
43. Never discuss unsatisfactory test results with a patient unless the doctor directs you to do so.		
44. Medical assistants are not allowed to take care of prescription refill requests.		

PSY TRIAGE

Grade: ____________

45. Triage the following calls by writing the letters in the proper order. ____________________

a. Line 1: A school nurse calls with a question about a medical form.

b. Line 2: A mother calls about her child who is having an asthma attack.

c. Line 3: A father calls with a question about his daughter's medication.

d. Line 4: A patient calls complaining about a sore throat.

COG SHORT ANSWER

Grade: ____________

46. A woman calls the office frantic because she thinks she is having a heart attack. What information should you try to get first from the caller?

____

____

____

____

47. A patient in your office is having trouble breathing. You have been asked to call EMS. What five pieces of information will you need before you make the call?

____

____

____

____

48. Dr. Porter is in a meeting, but he has instructed you to communicate with him via cell phone when you get the test results back for a certain patient. However, he does not like to have his cell phone ring while he is in meetings. How will you communicate with him?

____

____

____

____

49. It is an exceptionally hot day in the spring. Because the air conditioner is not on yet, you take a chair from the waiting room and prop the door open with it. You also move the boxes that were delivered earlier away from the window so the air comes in. How is this a violation of the Americans with Disabilities Act?

____

____

____

____

50. You receive a call from a patient who complains of being short of breath. What questions will you ask to determine whether this is an emergency?

____

____

____

____

AFF PSY ACTIVE LEARNING

Grade: ____________

51. Working with two classmates, role-play a medical emergency in the physician's office waiting room. Have one person play the role of the patient, the second person play the role of the receptionist, and the third person play the role of the EMS call operator. The patient should describe his or her condition, and the receptionist is responsible for conveying these details to EMS. Switch roles so that everyone gets a chance to play each role.

AFF WHAT WOULD YOU DO?

Grade: ____________

52. Your office shows videos about healthy living, exercise, and nutrition throughout the day. It seems that most of the adults watch and enjoy the programming. One crowded afternoon, a patient comes up to the desk to complain that the programming is distracting and he would prefer having the television turned off. However, there are people in the room watching the television. What would you say to the upset patient?

____

____

____

____

53. Mrs. Gonzalez calls to schedule her annual checkup. She is put on hold, and when the receptionist comes back to her call, she is upset that she was placed on hold. When she comes in for her appointment, she says that the receptionist should deal with every call individually and that no one should be placed on hold. How would you explain the phone call triage system to her?

____

____

____

____

AFF CASE STUDY FOR CRITICAL THINKING

Grade: ___________

You are working for a pediatrician. A mother arrives carrying an 18-month-old child with symptoms of a respiratory illness. You ask for her insurance card and she yells, "take care of my child first." You are willing to rearrange the usual order of things, but when you direct her to sit in the sick-child area, as per office protocol, the mother refuses, stating, "I don't want my child to get sicker." Circle the appropriate response from the lists below each question.

54. What might you say to make the mother give you the insurance information?

- **a.** I am required to update your chart, including your insurance information, at each visit *before* you see the physician.
- **b.** The physician will not see your child until I see your card.
- **c.** You are being very difficult. Can we start over?
- **d.** I'll hold the child while you get your card out.

55. What is your best action regarding the waiting area?

- **a.** Tell the physician.
- **b.** Calmly explain the policy and why you have it.
- **c.** Even though you will be putting her ahead of others, put the child in an open exam room.
- **d.** Ask the mother to leave.
- **e.** Tell her to take the child to the emergency room.

56. What is the most important thing you can do to make difficult situations like this better?

- **a.** Place signs in the waiting area about behavior.
- **b.** Make sure your work area is clean and neat.
- **c.** Make sure you always have someone else with you in the reception area.
- **d.** Remain calm and act professionally.
- **e.** Stand your ground with the angry person.

PSY PROCEDURE 5-1 Handling Incoming Calls

Name: ______________________ Date: __________ Time: __________ Grade: __________

EQUIPMENT/SUPPLIES: Telephone, telephone message pad, writing utensil (pen or pencil), headset (if applicable)

STANDARDS: Given the needed equipment and a place to work, the student will perform this skill with ______% accuracy in a total of ______ minutes. *(Your instructor will tell you what the percentage and time limits will be before you begin.)*

KEY: 4 = Satisfactory 0 = Unsatisfactory NA = this step is not counted

PROCEDURE STEPS	SELF	PARTNER	INSTRUCTOR
1. Gather the needed equipment.	☐	☐	☐
2. Answer the phone within two rings.	☐	☐	☐
3. Greet caller with proper identification (your name and the name of the office).	☐	☐	☐
4. Identify the nature or reason for the call in a timely manner.	☐	☐	☐
5. Triage the call appropriately.	☐	☐	☐
6. Communicate in a professional manner and with unhurried speech.	☐	☐	☐
7. Clarify information as needed.	☐	☐	☐
8. Record the message on a message pad. Include the name of caller, date, time, telephone number where the caller can be reached, description of the caller's concerns, and person to whom the message is routed.	☐	☐	☐
9. Give the caller an approximate time for a return call.	☐	☐	☐
10. Ask the caller whether he or she has any additional questions or needs any other help.	☐	☐	☐
11. Allow the caller to disconnect first.	☐	☐	☐
12. Put the message in an assigned place.	☐	☐	☐
13. Complete the task within 10 minutes.	☐	☐	☐
14. AFF Explain how you would respond to a patient who is obviously angry.	☐	☐	☐

____

____

____

____

CALCULATION

Total Possible Points: ______

Total Points Earned: ______ Multiplied by 100 = ______ Divided by Total Possible Points = ______ %

PASS **FAIL** **COMMENTS:**

☐ ☐

Student's signature ______________________________ Date ______

Partner's signature ______________________________ Date ______

Instructor's signature ______________________________ Date ______

PSY PROCEDURE 5-2 Calling Emergency Medical Services

Name: __________________ Date: ________ Time: ________ Grade: ________

EQUIPMENT/SUPPLIES: Telephone, patient information, writing utensil (pen, pencil)

STANDARDS: Given the needed equipment and a place to work, the student will perform this skill with ______% accuracy in a total of ______ minutes. *(Your instructor will tell you what the percentage and time limits will be before you begin.)*

KEY: 4 = Satisfactory 0 = Unsatisfactory NA = this step is not counted

PROCEDURE STEPS	SELF	PARTNER	INSTRUCTOR
1. Obtain the following the information before dialing: patient's name, age, sex, nature of medical condition, type of service the physician is requesting, any special instructions or requests the physician may have, your location, and any special information for access.	☐	☐	☐
2. Dial 911 or other EMS number.	☐	☐	☐
3. Calmly provide the dispatcher with the above information.	☐	☐	☐
4. Answer the dispatcher's questions calmly and professionally.	☐	☐	☐
5. Follow the dispatcher's instructions, if applicable.	☐	☐	☐
6. End the call as per dispatcher instructions.	☐	☐	☐
7. Complete the task within 10 minutes.	☐	☐	☐
8. AFF Explain how you would respond to a family member who is getting in the way of performing this task.	☐	☐	☐

CALCULATION

Total Possible Points: ______

Total Points Earned: ______ Multiplied by 100 = ______ Divided by Total Possible Points = ______ %

PASS ☐ **FAIL** ☐ **COMMENTS:**

Student's signature ______________________ Date ______

Partner's signature ______________________ Date ______

Instructor's signature ______________________ Date ______

PSY PROCEDURE 5-3 Explain General Office Policies

Name: ____________________ Date: ________ Time: ________ Grade: ________

EQUIPMENT/SUPPLIES: Patient's chart, office brochure

STANDARDS: Given the needed equipment and a place to work, the student will perform this skill with ______% accuracy in a total of ______ minutes. *(Your instructor will tell you what the percentage and time limits will be before you begin.)*

KEY: 4 = Satisfactory 0 = Unsatisfactory NA = this step is not counted

PROCEDURE STEPS	SELF	PARTNER	INSTRUCTOR
1. Assess the patient's level of understanding.	☐	☐	☐
2. Review important areas and highlight these in the office brochure.	☐	☐	☐
3. Ask the patient if he or she understands or has any questions.	☐	☐	☐
4. Give the patient the brochure to take home.	☐	☐	☐
5. Put in place a procedure for updating information and letting patients know of changes.	☐	☐	☐
6. AFF Explain how you would instruct a hearing-impaired patient about office procedures.	☐	☐	☐

CALCULATION

Total Possible Points: ______

Total Points Earned: ______ Multiplied by 100 = ______ Divided by Total Possible Points = ______ %

PASS ☐ **FAIL** ☐ **COMMENTS:**

Student's signature ______________________________ Date ______

Partner's signature ______________________________ Date ______

Instructor's signature ______________________________ Date ______

CHAPTER

6 Managing Appointments

Learning Outcomes

Cognitive Domain

1. Spell and define the key terms
2. Describe the pros and cons of various types of appointment management systems for scheduling patient office visits, including manual and computerized scheduling
3. Describe scheduling guidelines
4. Explain guidelines for scheduling appointments for new patients, return visits, inpatient admissions, and outpatient procedures
5. Recognize office policies and protocols for handling appointments
6. Identify critical information required for scheduling patient admissions and/or procedures
7. Discuss referral process for patients in a managed care program
8. List three ways to remind patients about appointments
9. Describe how to triage patient emergencies, acutely ill patients, and walk-in patients
10. Describe how to handle late patients
11. Explain what to do if the physician is delayed
12. Describe how to handle patients who miss their appointments
13. Describe how to handle appointment cancellations made by the office or by the patient

Psychomotor Domain

1. Manage appointment schedule, using established priorities
   a. Schedule an appointment for a new patient (Procedure 6-1)
   b. Schedule an appointment for a return visit (Procedure 6-2)
2. Schedule patient admissions and/or procedures
   a. Schedule an appointment for a referral to an outpatient facility (Procedure 6-3)
   b. Arrange for admission to an inpatient facility (Procedure 6-4)
      - Verify eligibility for managed care services
      - Obtain precertification, including documentation
      - Apply third-party managed care policies and procedures
      - Apply third-party guidelines
3. Use office hardware and software to maintain office systems

Affective Domain

1. Implement time management principles to maintain effective office functions
2. Demonstrate empathy in communicating with patients, family, and staff
3. Demonstrate sensitivity in communicating with both providers and patients

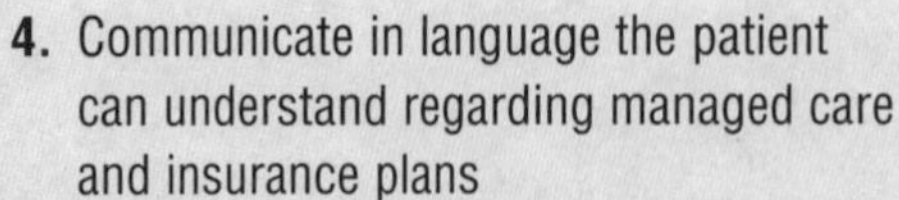

4. Communicate in language the patient can understand regarding managed care and insurance plans
5. Demonstrate recognition of the patient's level of understanding in communications

ABHES Competencies

1. Schedule and manage appointments
2. Schedule inpatient and outpatient admissions
3. Be impartial and show empathy when dealing with patients
4. Apply third-party guidelines
5. Obtain managed care referrals and precertification
6. Apply computer application skills using a variety of different electronic programs including both practice management software and EMR software
7. Communicate on the recipient's level of comprehension
8. Serve as liaison between physician and others

Name: ______________________ Date: __________ Grade: __________

COG MULTIPLE CHOICE

1. If your medical office uses a manual system of scheduled appointments for patient office visits, you will need a(n):
   a. toolbar.
   b. appointment book.
   c. computer.
   d. buffer time.
   e. fixed schedule.

2. How much time should be blocked off each morning and afternoon to accommodate emergencies, late arrivals, and other delays?
   a. 5 to 10 minutes
   b. 10 to 20 minutes
   c. 15 to 30 minutes
   d. 45 minutes to 1 hour
   e. 1 to 2 hours

3. When scheduling an appointment, why should you ask the patient the reason he or she needs to see the doctor?
   a. To know the level of empathy to give the patient.
   b. To anticipate the time needed for the appointment.
   c. To confront the patient about his or her personal choices.
   d. To manipulate the patient's needs.
   e. To determine who should see the patient.

4. Which of the following is an advantage to clustering?
   a. Efficient use of employee's time
   b. Increased patient time for the physician
   c. Reduced staff costs for the office
   d. Shorter patient appointments
   e. Greater need for specialists in the office

5. In fixed scheduling, the length of time reserved for each appointment is determined by the:
   a. physician's personal schedule.
   b. number of hours open on a given day.
   c. reason for the patient's visit.
   d. type of insurance provider.
   e. patient's age.

6. Double booking works well when patients are being sent for diagnostic testing because:
   a. it gives each patient enough time to prepare for testing.
   b. it leaves time to see both patients without keeping either one waiting unnecessarily.
   c. the physician enjoys seeing two patients at one time.
   d. it challenges the medical practice's resources.
   e. it gives the physician more "downtime."

7. Which of the following is a disadvantage to open hours?
   a. Patients with emergencies cannot be seen quickly.
   b. Scheduling patients is a challenge.
   c. Effective time management is almost impossible.
   d. Walk-ins are encouraged.
   e. Patient charts aren't properly updated.

8. You should leave some time slots open during the schedule each day to:
   a. allow patients to make their own appointments online.
   b. make the schedule more well rounded.
   c. leave some time for personal responsibilities.
   d. provide the staff some flex time.
   e. make room for emergencies and delays.

9. Most return appointments are made:

   a. before the patient leaves the office.
   b. before the patient's appointment.
   c. after the patient leaves the office.
   d. during the patient's next visit.
   e. when the patient receives a mailed reminder.

10. Reminder cards should be mailed:

   a. the first day of every month.
   b. a week before the date of the appointment.
   c. the beginning of the year.
   d. with all billing statements.
   e. only when the patient requests one.

11. A condition that is abrupt in onset is described as:

   a. chronic.
   b. commonplace.
   c. lethal.
   d. acute.
   e. incurable.

12. Who is authorized to make the decision whether to see a walk-in patient or not?

   a. Medical assistant
   b. Emergency medical technician
   c. Provider
   d. Reception
   e. Nurse

13. If you reschedule an appointment, you should note the reason for the cancellation or rescheduling in:

   a. the patient's chart.
   b. the patient's immunization record.
   c. the patient's insurance card.
   d. the patient's billing form.
   e. the office's appointment book.

14. If you have to cancel on the day of an appointment because of a physician's illness:

   a. send the patient an apology letter.
   b. give the patient a detailed excuse.
   c. e-mail the patient a reminder.
   d. call the patient and explain.
   e. offer the patient a discount at his or her next appointment.

15. If you find that your schedule is chaotic nearly every day, then you should:

   a. evaluate the schedule over time.
   b. keep that information private.
   c. tell your supervisor that you would like a new job.
   d. stop the old schedule and make a new one.
   e. let the patients know that the schedule isn't working.

16. An instruction to transfer a patient's care to a specialist is a:

   a. precertification.
   b. consultation.
   c. transfer.
   d. referral.
   e. payback.

17. Established patients are:

   a. patients who are new to the practice.
   b. patients who have been to the practice before.
   c. patients who are over age 65 years.
   d. patients who are chronically ill.
   e. patients with insurance.

18. A flexible scheduling method that schedules patients for the first 30 minutes of an hour and leaves the second half of each hour open is called:

   a. clustering.
   b. wave scheduling system.
   c. streaming.
   d. fixed-schedule system.
   e. double booking.

19. A chronic problem is one that is:

a. not very serious.

b. occurring for a short period of time.

c. longstanding.

d. easily cured.

e. difficult to diagnose.

20. Which of the following is true of a constellation of symptoms?

a. It can only be assessed by a physician.

b. It is only an emergency if a patient is having a heart attack.

c. It means a patient is suffering from appendicitis.

d. It is a group of clinical signs indicating a particular disease.

e. It probably requires a call to emergency medical services.

21. When a patient calls with an emergency, your first responsibility is to:

a. determine if the patient has an appointment.

b. decide whether the problem can be treated in the office.

c. verify that the physician can see the patient.

d. identify the patient's constellation of symptoms.

22. What should you do if the physician decides not to see a walk-in patient?

a. Ask the patient to schedule an appointment to return later.

b. Explain that the physician is too busy.

c. Tell the patient to try a different medical office.

d. Tell the patient to go to the hospital.

23. When might you write a letter to a patient who has an appointment that you must cancel?

a. when you can't reach the patient by phone

b. when the physician leaves the office abruptly

c. when you do not have the patient's demographic information

d. when you want to use written communication

COG MATCHING

Grade: ______

Match the following key terms to their definitions.

Key Terms	Definitions
24. ______ acute	a. a group of clinical signs indicating a particular disease process
25. ______ buffer	b. the practice of booking two patients for the same period with the same physician
26. ______ chronic	c. term used in the medical field to indicate that something should be done immediately
27. ______ clustering	d. a system for blocking off unavailable patient appointment times
28. ______ constellation of symptoms	e. a flexible scheduling method that allows time for procedures of varying lengths and the addition of unscheduled patients, as needed
29. ______ consultation	f. referring to a longstanding medical problem
30. ______ double booking	g. grouping patients with similar problems or needs
31. ______ matrix	

32. _____ precertification
33. _____ providers
34. _____ referral
35. _____ STAT
36. _____ streaming
37. _____ wave scheduling system

h. a method of allotting time for appointments based on the needs of the individual patient that helps minimize gaps in time and backups
i. extra time booked on the schedule to accommodate emergencies, walk-ins, and other demands on the provider's daily time schedule that are not considered direct patient care
j. health care workers who deliver medical care
k. referring to a medical problem with abrupt onset
l. request for assistance from one physician to another
m. approved documentation prior to referrals to specialists and other facilities
n. instructions to transfer a patient's care to a specialist

COG SHORT ANSWER

Grade: _____

38. List four advantages to clustering patients.

_____

_____

_____

_____

39. Name the three factors that can affect scheduling.

_____

_____

_____

_____

40. List the three ways to remind patients about appointments.

_____

_____

_____

_____

41. When calling another physician's office for an appointment for your patient, you'll need to provide certain information. List the seven pieces of information that you should provide to another physician's office.

---

42. List three items usually included in preadmission testing for surgery.

COG TRUE OR FALSE?

Grade: ______

Determine whether the following statements are true or false. If false, explain why.

43. Fixed scheduling is the most commonly used method.

---

44. A medical office that operates with open hours for patient visits is open 24 hours a day, 7 days a week.

---

45. Most appointments for new patients are made in person.

---

46. Patients with medical emergencies need to be seen immediately.

COG PSY ACTIVE LEARNING

Grade: ________

47. The appointment book below is divided into half-hour increments. The spaces below each time slot are empty. Fill in the appointment book with the following information: Dr. Brown has hospital rounds from 8:00 a.m. to 9:00 a.m. He has the following appointments: Cindy Wallis at 9:30 a.m.; Bill Waters at 10:00 a.m.; Rodney Kingston at 10:30 a.m.

8:00	8:30	9:00	9:30	10:00	10:30

Draw a line from the service to the appropriate time allotment.

Service	Estimated Time
48. blood pressure check	**a.** 5 minutes
49. complete physical exam	**b.** 10 minutes
50. dressing change	**c.** 15 minutes
51. recheck	**d.** 30 minutes
52. school physical	**e.** 1 hour

COG IDENTIFICATION

Grade: ________

Identify each type of scheduling system in the chart below.

Description	Type of Scheduling System
53. Several patients are scheduled for the first 30 minutes of each hour.	
54. Appointments are given based on the needs of individual patients.	
55. Each hour is divided into increments of 15, 30, 45, or 60 minutes for appointments depending on the reason for the visit.	
56. Patients are grouped according to needs or problems.	
57. Two patients are scheduled for the same period with the same physician.	

COG PSY CORRECT OR INCORRECT?

Grade: _______

Below are the steps for making a return appointment. Some of the steps are false or incomplete. Review each step and then decide if it is correct or incorrect. If incorrect, rewrite the statement to make it true and complete.

58. Carefully check your appointment book or screen before offering an appointment time. If a specific examination, test, or x-ray is to be performed on the return visit, avoid scheduling two patients for the same examination at the same time.

____

59. Ask the patient when he or she would like to return.

____

60. Write the patient's name and telephone number in the appointment book or enter the information in computer.

____

61. Transfer the information to an appointment card that you will mail out to the patient at a later date.

____

62. Double-check your book or screen to be sure there are no errors.

____

63. End your conversation with a pleasant word and a smile.

____

AFF WHAT WOULD YOU DO?

Grade: _______

64. An older adult patient walks into the medical office. His constellation of symptoms includes chest discomfort, shortness of breath, and nausea. He doesn't have an appointment. Explain what you would do.

____

____

____

____

65. Sometimes, a patient may neglect to keep an appointment. When this happens, you should call the patient. What should you do if you are unable to reach the patient by phone?

____

____

____

____

66. Maria has just called into the office to cancel her appointment for today. Explain what you should do.

____

____

____

____

67. If diagnostic testing requires preparation from the patient, what should you do?

____

____

____

____

AFF PATIENT EDUCATION

Grade: ________

68. Juan is consistently late for appointments. You've spoken with him several times. What should you do next? Explain what you will you say to him and the information you will provide him with.

____

____

____

____

AFF CASE STUDY FOR CRITICAL THINKING A

Grade: ________

You are the RMA at the front desk of a busy family practice. The success of the day depends on how smoothly the schedule runs. It is your responsibility to check patients in as they arrive. Your office uses a sign-in sheet. Mr. Simpson is always late for his appointments and today is no exception.

69. Regarding the sign-in sheet, what other methods could you use that would limit the potential for invasion of patient privacy?

a. Have patients give their name to the receptionist as they arrive.

b. Periodically walk through the waiting area to see who is there.

c. Post a sign asking patients to whisper when they speak.

d. Use a sign-in clipboard that has a sliding shield to prevent seeing other names.

70. You notice that patients typically wait 30 to 45 minutes past their scheduled appointment times because the physician is chronically behind schedule. How would you handle the situation? Circle the best answer.

a. Tell the office manager to talk to him or you will find other employment.

b. Ask the office manager to put the issue of running behind on the next office meeting agenda.

c. Ask to speak with him or her in private and explain how his running behind affects the entire office.

d. Tease him or her about running behind in front of the patients and employees.

71. Circle the best strategy to handle Mr. Simpson's chronic tardiness.

a. Schedule him for the last appointment of the day.

b. Dismiss him from the physician's care.

c. Call his family and ask if they can get him there on time.

d. Tell him that he is messing up your whole day and he MUST stop being late.

e. Do not worry about it. No matter what you do, he will still be late.

PSY PROCEDURE 6-1 Scheduling an Appointment for a New Patient

Name: ______________________ Date: __________ Time: __________ Grade: __________

EQUIPMENT/ITEMS NEEDED: Patient's demographic information, patient's chief complaint, appointment book or computer with appointment software, information found in Activity #1

STANDARDS: Given the needed equipment and a place to work the student will perform this skill with _______% accuracy in a total of __________ minutes. *(Your instructor will tell you what the percentage and time limits will be before you begin.)*

KEY: 4 = Satisfactory 0 = Unsatisfactory NA = This step is not counted

PROCEDURE STEPS	SELF	PARTNER	INSTRUCTOR
1. Obtain as much information as possible from the patient, such as: • Full name and correct spelling • Mailing address (not all offices require this) • Day and evening telephone numbers • Reason for the visit • Name of the referring person	☐	☐	☐
2. Determine the patient's chief complaint or the reason for seeing the physician.	☐	☐	☐
3. Explain the payment policy of the practice. Instruct patients to bring all pertinent insurance information.	☐	☐	☐
4. Give concise directions if needed.	☐	☐	☐
5. Ask the patient if it is permissible to call at home or at work.	☐	☐	☐
6. Confirm the time and date of the appointment.	☐	☐	☐
7. Check your appointment book to be sure that you have placed the appointment on the correct day in the right time slot.	☐	☐	☐
8. If the patient was referred by another physician, call that physician's office before the appointment for copies of laboratory work, radiology, pathology reports, and so on. Give this information to the physician prior to the patient's appointment.	☐	☐	☐
9. AFF Explain how you would respond in a situation in which a patient does NOT give permission to phone him or her at work.	☐	☐	☐

____

____

____

____

CALCULATION

Total Possible Points: ______

Total Points Earned: ________ Multiplied by 100 = ________ Divided by Total Possible Points = ________ %

PASS ☐ **FAIL** ☐ **COMMENTS:**

Student's signature ________________________________ Date ______

Partner's signature ________________________________ Date ______

Instructor's signature ________________________________ Date ______

PSY PROCEDURE 6-2 Scheduling an Appointment for an Established Patient

Name: ______________________ Date: __________ Time: __________ Grade: __________

EQUIPMENT: Appointment book or computer with appointment software, appointment card, information found in Activity #1

STANDARDS: Given the needed equipment and a place to work the student will perform this skill with ________% accuracy in a total of ________ minutes. *(Your instructor will tell you what the percentage and time limits will be before you begin.)*

KEY: 4 = Satisfactory 0 = Unsatisfactory NA = This step is not counted

PROCEDURE STEPS	SELF	PARTNER	INSTRUCTOR
1. Determine what will be done at the return visit. Check your appointment book or computer system before offering an appointment.	☐	☐	☐
2. Offer the patient a specific time and date. Avoid asking the patient when he or she would like to return, as this can cause indecision.	☐	☐	☐
3. Write the patient's name and telephone number in the appointment book or enter it in the computer.	☐	☐	☐
4. Transfer the pertinent information to an appointment card and give it to the patient. Repeat aloud the appointment day, date, and time to the patient as you hand over the card.	☐	☐	☐
5. Double-check your book or computer to be sure you have not made an error.	☐	☐	☐
6. End your conversation with a pleasant word and a smile.	☐	☐	☐
7. AFF Explain how you would respond to a patient who insists on coming for a return appointment at a time when their doctor is in surgery.	☐	☐	☐

____

____

____

____

CALCULATION

Total Possible Points: ______

Total Points Earned: ______ Multiplied by 100 = ______ Divided by Total Possible Points = ______ %

PASS **FAIL** **COMMENTS:**

☐ ☐

Student's signature ______________________ Date ______

Partner's signature ______________________ Date ______

Instructor's signature ______________________ Date ______

PSY PROCEDURE 6-3 Scheduling an Appointment for a Referral to an Outpatient Facility

Name: ______________________ Date: __________ Time: __________ Grade: __________

EQUIPMENT: Patient's chart with demographic information; physician's order for services needed by the patient and reason for the services; patient's insurance card with referral information, referral form, and directions to office, information found in Activity #3

STANDARDS: Given the needed equipment and a place to work, the student will perform this skill with ________% accuracy in a total of ________ minutes. *(Your instructor will tell you what the percentage and time limits will be before you begin.)*

KEY: 4 = Satisfactory 0 = Unsatisfactory NA = This step is not counted

PROCEDURE STEPS	SELF	PARTNER	INSTRUCTOR
1. Make certain that the requirements of any third-party payers are met.	☐	☐	☐
2. Refer to the preferred provider list for the patient's insurance company. Allow the patient to choose a provider from the list.	☐	☐	☐
3. Have the following information available when you make the call: • Physician's name and telephone number • Patient's name, address, and telephone number • Reason for the call • Degree of urgency • Whether the patient is being sent for consultation or referral	☐	☐	☐
4. Record in the patient's chart the time and date of the call and the name of the person who received your call.	☐	☐	☐
5. Tell the person you are calling that you wish to be notified if your patient does not keep the appointment. If this occurs, be sure to tell your physician and enter this information in the patient's record.	☐	☐	☐
6. Write down the name, address, and telephone number of the doctor you are referring your patient to and include the date and time of the appointment. Give or mail this information to your patient. Be certain that the information is complete, accurate, and easy to read.	☐	☐	☐
7. If the patient is to call the referring physician to make the appointment, ask the patient to call you with the appointment date, then document this in the chart.	☐	☐	☐
8. AFF Explain how you would handle the following situation: There are two physicians listed for a certain specialty in a patient's managed care's preferred provider list. The patient asks you who she should choose.	☐	☐	☐

CALCULATION

Total Possible Points: ______

Total Points Earned: ________ Multiplied by 100 = ________ Divided by Total Possible Points = ________ %

PASS **FAIL** **COMMENTS:**

☐ ☐

Student's signature ____ Date ______

Partner's signature ____ Date ______

Instructor's signature ____ Date ______

PSY PROCEDURE 6-4 Arranging for Admission to an Inpatient Facility

Name: ______________________ Date: __________ Time: __________ Grade: __________

EQUIPMENT: Physician's order with diagnosis, patient's chart with demographic information, contact information for inpatient facility, information found in Activity #2

STANDARDS: Given the needed equipment and a place to work, the student will perform this skill with ________% accuracy in a total of ________ minutes. *(Your instructor will tell you what the percentage and time limits will be before you begin.)*

KEY: 4 = Satisfactory 0 = Unsatisfactory NA = This step is not counted

PROCEDURE STEPS	SELF	PARTNER	INSTRUCTOR
1. Determine the place patient and/or physician wants the admission arranged.	☐	☐	☐
2. Gather information for the other facility, including demographic and insurance information.	☐	☐	☐
3. Determine any precertification requirements. If needed, locate contact information on the back of the insurance card and call the insurance carrier to obtain a precertification number.	☐	☐	☐
4. Obtain from the physician the diagnosis and exact needs of the patient for an admission.	☐	☐	☐
5. Call the admissions department of the inpatient facility and give information from step 2.	☐	☐	☐
6. Obtain instructions for the patient and call or give the patient instructions and information.	☐	☐	☐
7. Provide the patient with the physician's orders for their hospital stay, including diet, medications, bed rest, etc.	☐	☐	☐
8. Document time, place, etc. in patient's chart, including any precertification requirements completed.	☐	☐	☐
9. AFF Explain how you would respond to a patient who is visibly shaken about finding out that he is being admitted to the hospital.	☐	☐	☐

____

____

____

____

CALCULATION

Total Possible Points: ______

Total Points Earned: ________ Multiplied by 100 = ________ Divided by Total Possible Points = ________ %

PASS **FAIL** **COMMENTS:**

☐ ☐

Student's signature ________________________________ Date ______

Partner's signature ________________________________ Date ______

Instructor's signature ________________________________ Date ______

Activity #1: Scheduling New and Returning Patients

Place the patients on the appointment book page provided. In order to make this activity more realistic, imagine that the patients are calling the office in the order they are listed. You will need to determine the time needed for the visit and the urgency of the patient's problem in assigning slots. Refer to Box 6-1 in the textbook for suggested time allotment.

Set up the page and establish the matrix: Providers and availability:

Dr. Jones sees patients from 2:00 p.m. to 5:00 p.m. In surgery until 12:00.
Dr. Smith sees patients from 8:00 a.m. to 3:00 p.m. No lunch.
Dr. Stowe sees patients from 8:00 a.m. to 5:00 p.m. with lunch from 12:00-1:30 p.m.

Jessica Marshall, CMA (AAMA), can give injections and do blood pressure checks. Lunch 1:00-2:00 p.m. Use the lab column for patients who can see her.

Patient Name	Reason	Telephone #
1. Jeremy Cole	Stepped on rusty nail	570-7890
2. Cheryl Jennings (New)	Needs college physical	765-9087
3. Patty Cook	Sore throat	799-7225
4. Susan Stills	Woke up feeling dizzy	836-8765
5. Pamela Jones (New)	Wants to talk about weight reduction	765-0123
6. Steve Elliott	Hand laceration at work. (supv. called)	799-4391
7. Amy Quarrels	Vomiting and diarrhea × 3 days	571-5923
8. Layla Harris	Nosebleed that won't stop	799-0127
9. Sharon Morris	Needs refill on pain meds	836-2100
10. Jared Davis	Blood pressure check	792-8333
11. Ginger Parks	Knee injury last week, still swelling	791-4752
12. Landon Smythe	Coughing up blood	414-6787
13. Raymond Gray	Confused and foggy, per son	922-8641
14. Seth Etchison	Skin rash	266-0999
15. Raji Omar	Allergy injection	607-9125
16. Marilyn Easley	Shortness of breath and nausea	903-8957
17. Stephanie Lewis	Freq. urination and burning	792-1480
18. Shannon Mitchell	Pregnancy test	799-0731
19. Shantina Branch (New)	Kindergarten physical	792-4500
20. Lee Davis	Recheck on strep throat	799-4800

What might you do differently with the new patients?

___

___

___

___

THURSDAY, APRIL 11

HOUR		Dr. Jones	Dr. Smith	Dr. Stowe	Lab
8	00				
8	15				
8	30				
8	45				
9	00				
9	15				
9	30				
9	45				
10	00				
10	15				
10	30				
10	45				
11	00				
11	15				
11	30				
11	45				
12	00				
12	15				
12	30				
12	45				
1	00				
1	15				
1	30				
1	45				
2	00				
2	15				
2	30				
2	45				
3	00				
3	15				
3	30				
3	45				
4	00				
4	15				
4	30				
4	45				
5	00				
5	15				
5	30				
5	45				
6	00				
6	15				
6	30				
6	45				
7	00				
NOTES					

Activity #2: Scheduling Inpatient Admission

You work for Dr. James Gibbs, whose office is at 102 South Hawthorne Road, Winston-Salem, NC 27103. The office phone number is 336-760-4216.

Stella Walker is a 42-year-old female patient with diabetes. She has Blue Cross Blue Shield of NC. Her date of birth is 5/6/64. Her subscriber ID# is 260-21-5612. Her group # is 26178. She is the policyholder.

Dr. Gibbs instructs you to arrange admission to Forsyth Medical Center for Stella Walker for tomorrow. Her admitting diagnosis is uncontrolled diabetes. Her insurance requires that you precertify her for this admission. The doctor gives you his written orders and instructs you to give them to the patient to hand carry to the hospital.

You call the insurance company using the phone number on the back of her insurance card. The insurance company gives you the precertification number 1238952-1 and tells you that she is certified to stay in the hospital for 3 days. She has a $100.00 co-pay for a hospital stay.

Complete the form provided.

Hospital Admission

Patient Name: ______________________________

Patient Insurance Company: ______________________________

Patient Date of Birth: ______________________________

Patient Subscriber ID#: ______________________________

Patient Group #: ______________________________

Insurance Policy Holder: ______________________________

Precertification #: ______________________________

Reason for Admission: ______________________________

____

Admitting Physician Name and Address ______________________________

____

Approved Length of Stay: ______________________________

In-Patient Co-Pay: ______________________________

Activity #3: Scheduling an Outpatient Procedure

Using the information on the physician's order below, records the dates and times for appointments made for Grace Woods to have arthroscopy of the left knee and physical therapy at Miracle Rehabilitation before and after surgery. Read the information carefully!

Physician's Order:

Hinged knee brace fitting for use after surgery at Miracle Rehabilitation.

Left knee arthroscopy with medial meniscal repair. Follow up with me in office 5 days post op.

Physical Therapy at Miracle Rehabilitation for eight sessions beginning 1 week after surgery.

Date of surgery: ______________________

Date of Miracle Rehab appointment for fitting of brace: ______________________

Dates of Miracle Rehab physical therapy appointments: ______________________

____

____

Date of postoperative visit in your office: ______________________

CHAPTER 7

Written Communications

Learning Outcomes

Cognitive Domain

1. Spell and define the key terms
2. Recognize elements of fundamental writing skills
3. Discuss the basic guidelines for grammar, punctuation, and spelling in medical writing
4. Organize technical informaton and summaries
5. Discuss the 11 key components of a business letter
6. Describe the process of writing a memorandum
7. List the items that must be included in an agenda
8. Identify the items that must be included when typing minutes
9. Cite the various services available for sending written information
10. Discuss the various mailing options
11. Identify the types of incoming written communication seen in a physician's office
12. Explain the guidelines for opening and sorting mail
13. Discuss applications of electronic technology in effective communication

Psychomotor Domain

1. Compose a professional/business letter (Procedure 7-1)
2. Open and sort mail (Procedure 7-2)

Affective Domain

1. Use language/verbal skills that enable patient's understanding
2. Demonstrate empathy in communicating with patients, family, and staff
3. Demonstrate sensitivity appropriate to the message being delivered
4. Demonstrate recognition of the patient's level of understanding in communications

ABHES Competencies

1. Perform fundamental writing skills including correct grammar, spelling, and formatting techniques when writing prescriptions, documenting medical records, etc.
2. Apply electronic technology
3. Adapt communications to individual's ability to understand
4. Respond to and initiate written communications
5. Utilize electronic technology to receive, organize, prioritize, and transmit information
6. Use correct grammar, spelling, and formatting techniques in written word

Name: ______________________ Date: ____________ Grade: ____________

COG MULTIPLE CHOICE

Choose the letter preceding the correct answer.

1. In a letter, the word "Enc." indicates the presence of a(n):
   a. summary.
   b. abstract.
   c. enclosure.
   d. review.
   e. invitation.

2. If you are instructed to write using the semiblock format, then you should:
   a. indent the first line of each paragraph.
   b. use left justification for everything.
   c. use right justification for the date only.
   d. write the recipient's full name in the salutation.
   e. indent the first line of the first paragraph.

3. Which of the following items can be abbreviated in an inside address?
   a. City
   b. Town
   c. Recipient's name
   d. Business title
   e. State

4. Which sentence is written correctly?
   a. "We will have to do tests" said Doctor Mathis, "Then we will know what is wrong."
   b. "We will have to do tests" said Doctor Mathis. "Then we will know what is wrong."
   c. "We will have to do tests," said Doctor Mathis "Then we will know what is wrong."
   d. "We will have to do tests", said Doctor Mathis "Then we will know what is wrong."
   e. "We will have to do tests," said Doctor Mathis. "Then we will know what is wrong."

5. Which term should be capitalized?
   a. morphine
   b. fluoxetine
   c. zithromax
   d. antibiotic
   e. catheter

6. If the fax machine is busy when sending an important fax, you should:
   a. mail the document instead.
   b. call the recipient and ask him to contact you when the machine is available.
   c. ask a coworker to send the document.
   d. make a note in the patient's chart.
   e. wait with the document until you receive confirmation that it was sent.

7. Which sentence is written correctly?
   a. The patient is 14 years old and is urinating 3 times more than normal.
   b. The patient is 14 years old and is urinating three times more than normal.
   c. The patient is fourteen years old and is urinating 3 times more than normal.
   d. The patient is fourteen years old and is urinating three times more than normal.
   e. The patient is fourteen years old and is urinating three times more than normally.

8. Which of the following always belongs on a fax cover sheet?
   a. The number of pages, not including the cover sheet
   b. A confidentiality statement
   c. A summary of the content of the message
   d. A summary of the content of the message, less confidential portions
   e. The name of the patient discussed in the message

9. The USPS permit imprint program:

a. guarantees overnight delivery.
b. provides receipt of delivery.
c. offers physicians cheaper postage.
d. deducts the postage charges from a prepaid account.
e. addresses envelopes for no additional charge.

10. Which USPS service will allow you to send a parcel overnight?

a. Registered mail
b. First-class mail
c. Presorted mail
d. Priority mail
e. Express mail

11. Which is the best way to highlight a list of key points in a business letter?

a. Use boldface text.
b. Use a larger font.
c. Use bulleted text.
d. Use a highlighter.
e. Use italicized text.

Scenario for questions 12-14: You are tasked with writing a letter to a patient on the basis of a chart from his last visit. Most important is a diagnosis listed as "HBV infection."

12. Which is an appropriate course of action?

a. Including the words "HBV infection" in the letter
b. Consulting the physician on the meaning of the term
c. Omitting the diagnosis from the otherwise complete letter
d. Guessing the meaning of the term and writing about that
e. Asking the office manager what to do about the letter

13. Having learned that HBV means hepatitis B virus, you should:

a. research HBV infection.
b. give the patient your condolences.
c. write a letter based on the physician's instructions.
d. immediately schedule an appointment for the patient.
e. ask the patient to visit the office to learn his or her condition.

14. Who might receive a memorandum you have written?

a. A nurse in your office
b. A drug sales representative
c. An insurance agent
d. An outside specialist
e. A recently admitted patient

15. Which closing is written correctly?

a. Best Regards
b. Sincerely Yours,
c. Best regards,
d. Sincerely yours
e. Best Regards,

16. The purpose of an agenda is to:

a. summarize the opinions expressed at a meeting.
b. provide a brief outline for topics to be discussed at a meeting.
c. inform participants of any changes since the last meeting.
d. remind group members about an upcoming meeting.
e. communicate key issues that should be addressed at future meetings.

17. Correspondence that contains information about a patient should be marked:
    - a. personal.
    - b. confidential.
    - c. urgent.
    - d. classified.
    - e. top secret.

18. Which of these should be included in minutes?
    - a. Individuals' statements
    - b. Your opinion of the vote
    - c. Names of those voting against
    - d. Names of those voting in favor
    - e. Date and time of the next meeting

19. Which type of mail provides the greatest protection for valuables?
    - a. Certified mail
    - b. International mail
    - c. Registered mail
    - d. Standard mail
    - e. First class mail

20. Among these, which type of mail should be handled first?
    - a. Medication samples
    - b. Professional journals
    - c. Insurance information
    - d. Patient correspondence
    - e. Waiting room magazines

21. Which charting note is written correctly?
    - a. Patient is a forty-four-year-old Hispanic man with two sprained fingers.
    - b. Patient is a 44-year-old hispanic man with 2 sprained fingers.
    - c. Patient is a 44-year-old Hispanic man with 2 sprained fingers.
    - d. Patient is a 44-year-old hispanic man with two sprained fingers.

22. Which of these statements is both clear and concise?
    - a. Mr. Jensen entered the office in the early evening complaining of stomach pain unlike any he had felt before.
    - b. Mr. Jensen complained of severe stomach pain.
    - c. Mr. Jensen came to the office complaining about pain.
    - d. Mr. Jensen complained about stomach pain before leaving the office.

COG MATCHING

Grade: _________

Match the following key terms to their definitions.

Key Terms	Definitions
23. _____ agenda	a. an informal intra-office communication, generally used to make brief announcements
24. _____ annotation	b. a typographic style
25. _____ BiCaps/intercaps	c. a type of letter format in which the first sentence is indented
26. _____ block	d. additional information intended to highlight key points in a document, typically written in margins
27. _____ enclosure	e. the process of reading a text to check grammatical and factual accuracy
28. _____ font	

29. _____ full block
30. _____ margin
31. _____ memorandum
32. _____ proofread
33. _____ salutation
34. _____ semiblock
35. _____ template
36. _____ transcription

f. a model used to ensure consistent format in writing
g. abbreviations, words, or phrases with unusual capitalization
h. a type of letter format in which all letter components are justified left
i. something that is included with a letter
j. the process of typing a dictated message
k. a brief outline of the topics discussed at a meeting
l. a type of letter format in which the date, subject line, closing, and signatures are justified right, and all other lines are justified left
m. the greeting of a letter
n. the blank space around the edges of a piece of paper that has been written on

SHORT ANSWER

Grade: _____

37. List the items that are usually included in the minutes of a business meeting.

_____

_____

_____

38. What three things must be included on every piece of mail before sending it?

_____

_____

_____

39. Why is an agenda useful for meetings? What does it include?

_____

_____

_____

40. What should you do after composing a piece of written communication? Why?

_____

_____

_____

AFF WHAT WOULD YOU DO?

Grade: ________

41. Suppose the physician told you to read his e-mails while he was on vacation. In doing so, you come across a personal piece of information that you know he would not want you to see. How would you handle it? Would you tell anyone that you saw it? Would you question the physician about it?

____

____

____

PSY ACTIVE LEARNING

Grade: ________

42. Compose a letter from Dr. Joseph Cohen, 321 Gasthaus Lane, Germantown, PA 87641, to Mr. Ligero Delgado, 888 La Sala Boulevard, Germantown, PA 87642.

The letter should inform Mr. Delgado of the following:

- The results of the biopsy taken during his sigmoidoscopy were negative.
- While these initial results are encouraging, his medical complaints need to be investigated further. Dr. Cohen would like to refer Mr. Delgado to a specialist, Dr. Douloureux.
- Dr. Douloureux's practice is in Suite 100 of the Atroce Medical Center, 132 West Broadway, Germantown, PA 87642.
- With Mr. Delgado's consent, his records can be forwarded to Dr. Douloureux and an appointment will be arranged.

Prepare the letter on a sheet of letterhead if available. If this is not available to you, print the letter on a standard 8 1/2 × 11 white paper and attach to this sheet. Proof your unedited copy and, using proofreader's marks, indicate your corrections. Make the corrections and reprint a final copy. Ask your instructor to review both copies.

43. Write 10 sentences using terms from Box 7-3. Use some terms correctly and others incorrectly. Exchange your sentences with another student. Correct your peer's sentences.

44. Collect five pieces of mail that you have received at home. What method of affixing postage did they use? Go to your local USPS office. Obtain either a priority mail or express mail envelope. Correctly address the envelope.

COG CORRECT OR INCORRECT?

Grade: ________

Read the following sentences. If the sentence is free of errors, write "correct" on the line. If the sentence contains errors, circle the problem and explain how you would fix the sentence.

45. The patient has a cold and is bothered by the postnasal drip.

____

46. The patient complained of constipation and has not had a bowl movement in 3 days.

____

47. The patient, Mrs. Philips, sought weight-loss advise from the physician.

____

48. The nurse applied antiseptic to the wounded elbow.

____

COG IDENTIFICATION

Grade: _______

Review the list of terms below and place a check mark to indicate whether each term must always be capitalized.

Name	Always	Not Always
49. Streptococcus		
50. Tylenol		
51. Benadryl		
52. Diagnosis		
53. Analgesic		
54. Merck		
55. Antihistamine		
56. Tampax		

COG PSY ACTIVE LEARNING

Grade: _______

57. Dr. Bruce Mosley asks you to prepare a memorandum for distribution to the entire office. He hands you a note to use as the body of the memo. It reads as follows:

On May 9, Jerry Henderson, a representative of Conrad Insurance, will be visiting the office during the morning. Please extend him the utmost courtesy and introduce yourself if you have not yet met him. Jerry is a wonderful man who has been very helpful to our practice. I will be unavailable during the morning as a result of his visit. Please direct questions to Shelly or Dr. Garcia. Of course, I may be contacted in case of an emergency. Using the sample memorandum format in Figure 7-5 of your text, construct the memo.

COG IDENTIFICATION

Grade: ________

58. You have been asked to send a summary of a patient's recent visit to a specialist. Review the list of forms of written communication below and place a check mark to indicate whether it is an appropriate means of written communication.

Form	Appropriate	Not Appropriate
a. A formal letter labeled confidential		
b. An e-mail marked *urgent*		
c. A memorandum		
d. A fax with a confidentiality statement		
e. A memorandum labeled *urgent*		

59. You always take the minutes at the staff meeting, but you'll be on vacation during the next meeting. Identify and list for your coworker what information belongs in the minutes.

____

____

____

60. Dr. Shadrick is at a week-long conference in another state. She needs a patient's complete history to present to the conference one day from now, but has forgotten it at the office. Name three suitable delivery options.

a. ____________________

b. ____________________

c. ____________________

61. Which of the following is/are good practice(s) in regard to handling mail? Place a check mark in the correct box below to answer "Yes" or "No."

Practice	Yes	No
a. Handling promotional materials last		
b. Opening mail addressed to a physician marked "confidential"		
c. Asking a physician or office manager about a piece of mail you are unsure about		
d. Leaving patient correspondence in an external mailbox		
e. Disposing of a physician's personal mail if he or she is away		
f. Informing a covering physician about mail requiring urgent attention		
g. Prioritizing patient care-related mail over pharmaceutical samples		

AFF PSY WHAT WOULD YOU DO?

Grade: _______

62. You are asked to open the mail today. There is a variety of material including several letters addressed to the physician marked "Urgent," "Confidential," and "Personal." Some of the other mail is from patients, but it is not marked in any unusual fashion. Other letters are from insurance companies with which your office is associated. There are also several advertisements and promotional mailings from medical supply companies, pharmaceutical companies, and insurance companies. In addition, there are pieces of mail that do not include a return address. Explain the procedure you would follow in dealing with this mail.

____

____

____

____

PSY PATIENT EDUCATION

Grade: _______

63. The office's policy is to mail a welcome letter to new patients. Make a list of information that should be included in this letter so the patient is prepared for her first visit.

____

____

____

____

AFF CASE STUDY FOR CRITICAL THINKING

Grade: ______

The office manager has asked you to compose a letter to every patient in the practice explaining why their physician will be out of the office for ten months. The physician is having extensive cosmetic surgery and is taking a medical leave of absence.

64. Your letter should _____ should not _____ include the reason for the absence.

65. Circle the more appropriate sentence for your letter from the two choices below:

a. This letter is to tell you that Dr. Smith will not be here for the next ten months, effective October 1, 2012.

b. This letter is to inform you that Dr. William Smith will be taking a ten-month leave of absence beginning October 1, 2012.

66. Circle the more appropriate sentence for your letter from the two choices below:

a. We hope you will continue to receive medical care from our office. We have 12 other providers who will be available to handle your health care needs.

b. Dr. Smith wants you to see one of our other many excellent providers in the interim.

PSY PROCEDURE 7-1 Composing a Business Letter

Name: ______________________ Date: __________ Time: __________ Grade: __________

EQUIPMENT/SUPPLIES: Computer with word processing software, 8 1/2 × 11 white paper, #10 sized envelope

STANDARDS: Given the needed equipment and a place to work, the student will perform this skill with ______ % accuracy in a total of ________ minutes. *(Your instructor will tell you what the percentage and time limits will be before you begin.)*

KEY: 4 = Satisfactory 0 = Unsatisfactory NA = This step is not counted

PROCEDURE STEPS	SELF	PARTNER	INSTRUCTOR
1. Move cursor down 2 lines below the letterhead and enter today's date, flush right.	☐	☐	☐
2. Flush left, move cursor down 2 lines and enter the inside address using the name and address of the person to whom you are writing.	☐	☐	☐
3. Double space and type the salutation followed by a colon.	☐	☐	☐
4. Enter a reference line.	☐	☐	☐
5. Double space between paragraphs.	☐	☐	☐
6. Double space and flush right, enter the complimentary close.	☐	☐	☐
7. Move cursor down 4 spaces and enter the sender's name.	☐	☐	☐
8. Double space and enter initials of the sender in all caps.	☐	☐	☐
9. Enter a slash and your initials in lower case letters.	☐	☐	☐
10. Enter c: and names of those who get copies of the letter.	☐	☐	☐
11. Enter Enc: and the number and description of each enclosed sheet.	☐	☐	☐
12. Print on letterhead.	☐	☐	☐
13. Proofread the letter.	☐	☐	☐
14. Attach the letter to the patient's chart.	☐	☐	☐
15. Submit to the sender of the letter for review and signature.	☐	☐	☐
16. Make a copy of the letter for the patient's chart.	☐	☐	☐
17. Address envelopes using all caps and no punctuation.	☐	☐	☐
18. AFF Explain how you would respond in this situation: your physician receives the letter you prepared and asks you to insert a comma where you know a comma is not required.	☐	☐	☐

____

____

____

____

CALCULATION

Total Possible Points: ______

Total Points Earned: ________ Multiplied by 100 = ________ Divided by Total Possible Points = ________ %

PASS ☐ **FAIL** ☐ **COMMENTS:**

Student's signature ____ Date ________

Partner's signature ____ Date ________

Instructor's signature ______________________________________ Date ________

PSY PROCEDURE 7-2 Opening and Sorting Incoming Mail

Name: ______________________ Date: __________ Time: __________ Grade: __________

EQUIPMENT/SUPPLIES: Letter opener, paper clips, directional tabs, date stamp

STANDARDS: Given the needed equipment and a place to work, the student will perform this skill with ______ % accuracy in a total of ______ minutes. *(Your instructor will tell you what the percentage and time limits will be before you begin.)*

KEY: 4 = Satisfactory 0 = Unsatisfactory NA = This step is not counted

PROCEDURE STEPS	SELF	PARTNER	INSTRUCTOR
1. Gather the necessary equipment.	☐	☐	☐
2. Open all letters and check for enclosures.	☐	☐	☐
3. Paper clip enclosures to the letter.	☐	☐	☐
4. Date-stamp each item.	☐	☐	☐
5. Sort the mail into categories and deal with it appropriately. Generally, you should handle the following types of mail as noted: *Correspondence regarding a patient:* **a.** Use a paper clip to attach letters, test results, etc. to the patient's chart. **b.** Place the chart in a pile for the physician to review. *Payments and other checks:* **a.** Record promptly all insurance payments and checks and deposit them according to office policy. **b.** Account for all drug samples and appropriately log them into the sample book.	☐	☐	☐
6. Dispose of miscellaneous advertisements unless otherwise directed.	☐	☐	☐
7. Distribute the mail to the appropriate staff members. For example, mail might be for the physician, nurse manager, office manager, billing clerk, or other personnel.	☐	☐	☐
8. AFF Explain how you would handle a letter marked "Personal and Confidential."	☐	☐	☐

____

____

____

____

CALCULATION

Total Possible Points: ______

Total Points Earned: ________ Multiplied by 100 = ________ Divided by Total Possible Points = ________ %

PASS **FAIL** **COMMENTS:**

☐ ☐

Student's signature ____ Date ________

Partner's signature ____ Date ________

Instructor's signature ____ Date ________

CHAPTER

8 Health Information Management and Protection

Learning Outcomes

Cognitive Domain

1. Spell and define the key terms
2. Explain the requirements of the Health Insurance Portability and Accountability Act relating to the sharing and saving of personal and protected health information
3. Identify types of records common to the health care setting
4. Describe standard and electronic health record systems
5. Explain the process for releasing medical records to third-party payers and individual patients
6. Discuss principles of using an electronic medical record
7. Describe various types of content maintained in a patient's medical record
8. Identify systems for organizing medical records
9. Explain how to make an entry in a patient's medical record, using abbreviations when appropriate
10. Explain how to make a correction in a standard and electronic health record
11. Discuss pros and cons of various filing methods
12. Describe indexing rules
13. Discuss filing procedures
14. Identify both equipment and supplies needed for filing medical records
15. Explain the guidelines of sound policies for record retention
16. Describe the proper disposal of paper and electronic protected health information (PHI)
17. Explore issue of confidentiality as it applies to the medical assistant
18. Describe the implications of HIPAA for the medical assistant in various medical settings

Psychomotor Domain

1. Establish, organize, and maintain a patient's medical record (Procedure 8-1)
2. File a medical record (Procedure 8-2)
3. Maintain organization by filing

Affective Domain

1. Demonstrate sensitivity to patient rights
2. Demonstrate awarenesss of the consequences of not working within the legal scope of practice
3. Recognize the importance of local, state and federal legislation and regulations in the practice setting
4. Respond to issues of confidentiality
5. Apply HIPAA rules in regard to privacy/release of information
6. Apply local, state and federal health care legislation and regulation appropriate to the medical assisting practice setting

ABHES Competencies

1. Perform basic clerical functions
2. Prepare and maintain medical records
3. Receive, organize, prioritize, and transmit information expediently
4. Apply electronic technology
5. Institute federal and state guidelines when releasing medical records or information
6. Efficiently maintain and understand different types of medical correspondence and medical reports

Name: ______________________ Date: __________ Grade: __________

COG MULTIPLE CHOICE

1. Who coordinates and oversees the various aspects of HIPAA compliance in a medical office?
   - a. Medicaid and Medicare
   - b. HIPAA officer
   - c. Privacy officer
   - d. Office manager
   - e. Law enforcement

2. A release of records request must contain the patient's:
   - a. next of kin.
   - b. home phone number.
   - c. original signature.
   - d. medical history.
   - e. date of birth.

3. Which is an example of protected health information?
   - a. Published statistics by a credible source
   - b. Insurance company's mailing address
   - c. Physician's pager number
   - d. First and last name associated with a diagnosis
   - e. Poll published in a medical journal

4. If patients believe their rights have been denied or their health information isn't being protected, they can file a complaint with the:
   - a. Journal of American Medical Assistants.
   - b. American Medical Association.
   - c. provider or insurer.
   - d. medical assistant.
   - e. state's attorney.

5. The only time an original record should be released is when the:
   - a. patient asks for the record.
   - b. patient is in critical condition.
   - c. record is subpoenaed by the court of law.
   - d. physician is being sued.
   - e. patient terminates the relationship with the physician.

6. Do medical records have the same content if they are on paper or a computer disk?
   - a. Yes
   - b. No
   - c. Sometimes
   - d. Most of the time
   - e. Never

7. Documentation of each patient encounter is called:
   - a. consultation reports.
   - b. medication administration.
   - c. correspondence.
   - d. narrative.
   - e. progress notes.

8. Improved medication management is a feature of:
   - a. SOAP.
   - b. electronic health records.
   - c. clearinghouses.
   - d. PHI.
   - e. workers' compensation.

9. To maintain security, a facility should:
   - a. design a written confidentiality policy for employees to sign.
   - b. provide public access to medical records.
   - c. keep a record of all passwords and give a copy to each employee.
   - d. keep doors unlocked during the evening hours only.
   - e. have employees hide patient information from other coworkers.

10. Under source-oriented records, the most recent documents are placed on top of previous sheets, which is called:

a. chronological order.

b. reverse chronological order.

c. alphabetical order.

d. subject order.

e. numeric order.

11. The acronym "SOAP" stands for:

a. subjective-objective-adjustment-plan.

b. subjective-objective-accounting-plan.

c. subjective-objective-assessment-plan.

d. subjective-objective-accounting-problem.

e. subjective-objective-assessment-problem.

12. The acronym "POMR" stands for:

a. presentation-oriented medical record.

b. protection-oriented medical record.

c. performance-oriented medical record.

d. professional-oriented medical record.

e. problem-oriented medical record.

13. Which of the following is contained in a POMR database?

a. Marketing tools

b. Field of interest

c. Job description

d. Review of systems

e. Accounting review

14. Which of the following will reflect each encounter with the patient chronologically, whether by phone, by e-mail, or in person?

a. Microfilm

b. Narrative

c. Progress notes

d. Subject filing

e. Flow sheet

15. Shingling is:

a. printing replies to a patient's e-mail.

b. recording laboratory results in the patient's chart.

c. telephone or electronic communications with patients.

d. taping the paper across the top to a regular-size sheet.

e. filing records in chronological order.

16. How long are workers' compensation cases kept open after the last date of treatment for any follow-up care that may be required?

a. 6 months

b. 1 year

c. 2 years

d. 5 years

e. 10 years

17. A cross-reference in numeric filing is called a(n):

a. open file.

b. locked file.

c. straight digit file.

d. master patient index.

e. duplication index.

18. Security experts advise storing backup disks:

a. in the office.

b. offsite.

c. at the physician's home.

d. on every computer.

e. at the library.

19. Drawer files are a type of:
    a. filing cabinet.
    b. storage container.
    c. computer system.
    d. shelving unit.
    e. subject filing.

20. The statute of limitations is:
    a. the end of a provider's ability to legally practice.
    b. the record retention system.
    c. a miniature photographic system.
    d. the legal time limit set for filing suit against an alleged wrongdoer.
    e. the number of records a storage system is able to hold.

COG MATCHING

Grade: ______

Match the following key terms to their definitions.

Key Terms

21. ____ alphabetic filing
22. ____ chief complaint
23. ____ chronological order
24. ____ clearinghouse
25. ____ covered entity
26. ____ cross-reference
27. ____ demographic data
28. ____ electronic health records (EHR)
29. ____ flow sheet
30. ____ medical history forms
31. ____ microfiche
32. ____ microfilm
33. ____ narrative
34. ____ numeric filing
35. ____ protected health information (PHI)
36. ____ present illness
37. ____ problem-oriented medical record (POMR)
38. ____ reverse chronological order
39. ____ SOAP
40. ____ subject filing

Definitions

a. information about patients that is recorded and stored on computer
b. photographs of records in a reduced size
c. a paragraph indicating the contact with the patient, what was done for the patient, and the outcome of any action
d. a specific account of the chief complaint, including time frames and characteristics
e. a common method of compiling information that lists each problem of the patient, usually at the beginning of the folder, and references each problem with a number throughout the folder
f. notation in a file indicating that a record is stored elsewhere and giving the reference; verification to another source; checking the tabular list against the alphabetic list in ICD-9 coding
g. entity that takes claims and other electronic data from providers, verifies the information, and forwards the proper forms to the payors for physicians
h. employer insurance for treatment of an employee's injury or illness related to the job
i. any information that can be linked to a specific person
j. items placed with oldest first
k. sheets of microfilm
l. arranging files according to their title, grouping similar subjects together
m. a style of charting that includes subjective, objective, assessment, and planning notes
n. arranging of names or titles according to the sequence of letters in the alphabet
o. health plan; health care clearinghouse; or health care provider who transmits any health information in electronic form in connection with a transaction covered under HIPAA
p. placing in order of time; usually the most recent is placed foremost

41. _____ workers' compensation

q. information relating to the statistical characteristics of populations

r. color-coded sheets that allow information to be recorded in graphic or tabular form for easy retrieval

s. arranging files by a numbered order

t. main reason for the visit to the medical office

u. record containing information about a patient's past and present health status

SHORT ANSWER

Grade: _____

42. List the four steps you should take to ensure that files are filed and retrieved quickly and efficiently.

43. Describe the difference between standard and electronic health record systems.

44. When documenting in a medical record or file, why should you use caution when using abbreviations?

45. How does a numeric filing system help a medical office meet HIPAA's privacy requirements?

46. Documentation is a large part of your job as a medical assistant. Legible, correct, and thorough documentation is necessary. List three instances, other than patient visits, when documentation is required.

47. When a health care provider's practice ends, either from retirement or death, what happens to the records?

48. Those who must abide by HIPAA are called "covered entities." List the three groups that are considered covered entities.

COG PSY ACTIVE LEARNING

Grade: ________________

49. If you were opening a new medical facility, consider whether you would want staff members using abbreviations in patient records. Then create a list of 20 acceptable abbreviations that may be used in your new facility. Next create a "Do Not Use" list for abbreviations that may be confusing and should not be included in records. Visit the website for the Joint Commission at www.jointcommission.org and include all of those abbreviations in addition to five other abbreviations of your own choice.

50. Interview a fellow student with a hypothetical illness. Document the visit with the chief complaint and history of present illness.

51. The office you work in receives lab results on a printer throughout the day. Write an office policy for maintaining confidentiality with the PHI being transmitted electronically.

52. Your medical office uses an alphabetic filing system. Place the following names in the correct order to show how you would place each record in a filing system.

Brandon P. Snow	Kristen F. Darian-Lewes	Shante L. Dawes	Emil S. Faqir, Jr.
Shaunice L. DeBlase	Juan R. Ortiz	Kim Soo	Fernando P. Vasquez, D.O.

a. ________________________________

b. ________________________________

c. ________________________________

d. ________________________________

e. ________________________________

f. ________________________________

g. ________________________________

h. ________________________________

COG IDENTIFICATION

Grade: ________________

53. HIPAA has privacy rules that protect your personal health information. Under HIPAA, covered entities must take certain safety measures to protect patients' information. Read the paragraph below. For each blank, there are two choices. Circle the correct word or phrase for each sentence.

Covered entities must designate a ________(a)________(HIPAA officer, privacy officer) to keep track of who has access to health information. They must also adopt written ________(b)________ (privacy, health care) procedures. Under HIPAA, patients have the right to decide if they provide ________(c)________ (permission, marketing) before their health information can be used or shared for certain purposes. They also have the right to get a ________(d)________ (narrative, report) on when and why their health care information was shared for certain purposes.

COG PSY IDENTIFICATION

Grade: ________

The rules for releasing medical records and authorization are meant to protect patients' privacy rights. Read the questions below regarding the release of medical records and circle "Yes" or "No" for each question.

54. May an 18-year-old patient get copies of his or her own medical records? Yes No

55. May all minors seek treatment for sexually transmitted diseases and birth control without parental knowledge or consent? Yes No

56. When a patient requests copies of his or her own records, does the doctor make the decision about what to copy? Yes No

57. Must the authorization form give the patient the opportunity to limit the information released? Yes No

58. When a patient authorizes the release of information, may he request that the physician leave out information pertinent to the situation? Yes No

COG FILL IN THE BLANKS

Grade: ________

HIPAA requirements provide guidelines and suggestions for safe computer practices when storing or transferring patient information. The following is a list of guidelines that medical facilities are urged to follow. Complete each sentence with the appropriate word from the word bank below.

59. Store ______________ in a bank safe-deposit box.

60. Change log-in ______________ and passwords every 30 days.

61. Turn ______________ away from areas where information may be seen by patients.

62. Use ______________ with ______________ other than letters.

63. Prepare a back-up ______________ for use when the computer system is down.

Word Bank

characters	plan	disks	information
codes	passwords	template	terminals

Note: Not all words will be used.

MATCHING

Grade: ______

A standard medical record in an outpatient facility, known as a chart or file, contains clinical information as well as billing and insurance information. In the clinical section of the file, you will often find certain types of information. In the columns below, draw a diagonal line to match the clinical type of information with its correct description.

Name of Clinical Information	Description
64. Chief complaint	**a.** Documentation of each patient encounter
65. Family and personal history	**b.** Provider's opinion of the patient's problem
66. Progress notes	**c.** Symptoms that led the patient to seek the physician's care
67. Diagnosis or medical impression	**d.** Letters or memos generated in the facility and sent out
68. Correspondence pertaining to patient	**e.** Review of major illnesses of family members

TRUE OR FALSE?

Grade: ______

69. True or False? Determine whether the following statements are true or false. If false, explain why.

a. HIPAA allows patients to ask to see and get a copy of their health records.

____

b. To maintain secure files, you should change log-in codes and passwords every 10 days.

____

c. Medical history forms are commonly used to gather information from the patient before the visit with the physician.

____

d. Before treating a patient for a possible workers' compensation case, you must first obtain verification from the employer unless the situation is life threatening.

____

AFF WHAT WOULD YOU DO?

Grade: _______

70. A mother is accused of physically abusing her 16-year-old daughter, a patient with your facility. A police officer who has been asked to investigate visits the medical office and asks for the patient's medical records. What would you do?

____

____

____

____

71. You're in the medical office and you suddenly realize that you've forgotten to document a telephone conversation you had with a patient 2 days ago. What would you do?

____

____

____

____

AFF CASE STUDY FOR CRITICAL THINKING A

Grade: ________

You are tasked with creating the office policy for the retention of records for your facility.

72. Circle any appropriate actions from the list below.

a. Research federal law that mandates how long you must keep records.

b. Research the state legislature to determine the statute of limitations for your state.

c. Make sure the time limit for retaining records includes inactive and closed files.

d. Set the time limits for retaining children's records from their 18th birthday.

e. Set the time limits for retaining the records of adults and children the same for ease of remembering.

f. Have the policy approved by the physician and/or appropriate employee.

73. This task is not in your job description, and you feel that you are not qualified to set policy for the facility. Circle the appropriate actions from the list below.

a. Tell your supervisor of your concerns and ask for his or her guidance.

b. Consider this a great opportunity to show your employer your skills.

c. Ask the attorney for the facility to create the policy for you.

d. Ask the attorney not to tell your supervisor that he helped you.

e. Do the task, but make sure everyone in the office knows who did it.

f. Do the task without assistance and ask for a promotion and/or raise when finished.

74. What is the statute of limitations for patients to file malpractice or negligence suits in your state? ____________

AFF CASE STUDY FOR CRITICAL THINKING B

Grade: _______

Your mother's best friend is a patient in the office where you work. You have known her all of your life. She has just been seen for a suspicious lump in her breast. She is very nervous and calls you at home that night to see if you know the results of her test. You saw the stat biopsy report before you left work and you know that the lump is malignant. She was given an appointment in 2 days for the physician to give her the results.

75. Circle all appropriate actions from the list below.

- **a.** Tell her that it is not in your scope of practice to give patients results without specific instructions from a provider, even if they are friends.
- **b.** To minimize the time she must anxiously wait, try to move her appointment to tomorrow as soon as you get to work in the morning.
- **c.** Tell her that the report was not good and to bring someone with her to the visit.
- **d.** Call the physician at home to ask if you can tell her.
- **e.** Tell her that you do not know the results of the test, but even if you did you could not tell her.
- **f.** Call your mother, tell her the situation, and ask for her advice.

76. Let's say you tell the patient that you cannot give test results, and she replies, "I have a right to know what is wrong with me." Circle all of the appropriate responses below.

- **a.** Only a provider can give test results in my office unless they specifically direct an employee to do so.
- **b.** I am a professional, and I don't really care about your rights.
- **c.** I know you are my mother's friend, but I am a CMA, and I follow the rules.
- **d.** Giving you the results of your biopsy may have caused me to get fired. I'm not getting fired for you or anybody.
- **e.** You do have that right, but I do not have the right to tell you.
- **f.** Talk to the physician about it.

77. Why is it important for the physician to give test results such as the one in the case study?

____

____

____

____

PSY PROCEDURE 8-1 Establishing, Organizing, and Maintaining a Medical File

Name: ______________________ Date: __________ Time: __________ Grade: __________

EQUIPMENT/SUPPLIES: File folder; metal fasteners; hole punch; five divider sheets with tabs, title, year, and alphabetic or numeric labels

STANDARDS: Given the needed equipment and a place to work the student will perform this skill with _______% accuracy in a total of _______ minutes. *(Your instructor will tell you what the percentage and time limits will be before you begin.)*

KEY: 4 = Satisfactory 0 = Unsatisfactory NA = this step is not counted

PROCEDURE STEPS	SELF	PARTNER	INSTRUCTOR
1. Place the label along the tabbed edge of the folder so that the title extends out beyond the folder itself. (Tabs can be either the length of the folder or tabbed in various positions, such as left, center, and right.)	☐	☐	☐
2. Place a year label along the top edge of the tab before the label with the title. This will be changed each year the patient has been seen. *Note:* Do not automatically replace these labels at the start of a new year; remove the old year and replace with a new one only when the patient comes in for the first visit of the new year.	☐	☐	☐
3. Place the appropriate alphabetic or numeric labels below the title.	☐	☐	☐
4. Apply any additional labels that your office may decide to use.	☐	☐	☐
5. Punch holes and insert demographic and financial information on the left side of the chart using top fasteners across the top.	☐	☐	☐
6. Make tabs for: Ex. H&P, Progress Notes, Medication Log, Correspondence, and Test Results.	☐	☐	☐
7. Place pages behind appropriate tabs.	☐	☐	☐
8. AFF Explain what you would do when you receive a revised copy correcting an error on a document already in a patient's chart.	☐	☐	☐

____

____

____

____

CALCULATION

Total Possible Points: ______

Total Points Earned: ______ Multiplied by 100 = ______ Divided by Total Possible Points = ______ %

PASS **FAIL** **COMMENTS:**

☐ ☐

Student's signature ________________________________ Date ______

Partner's signature ________________________________ Date ______

Instructor's signature ________________________________ Date ______

PSY

PROCEDURE 8-2 Filing Medical Records

Name: ______________________ Date: __________ Time: __________ Grade: __________

EQUIPMENT/SUPPLIES: Simulated patient file folder, several single sheets to be filed in the chart, file cabinet with other file

STANDARDS: Given the needed equipment and a place to work the student will perform this skill with ______% accuracy in a total of ______ minutes. *(Your instructor will tell you what the percentage and time limits will be before you begin.)*

KEY: 4 = Satisfactory 0 = Unsatisfactory NA = this step is not counted

PROCEDURE STEPS	SELF	PARTNER	INSTRUCTOR
1. Double check spelling of names on the chart and any single sheets to be placed in the folder.	☐	☐	☐
2. Condition any single sheets, etc.	☐	☐	☐
3. Place sheets behind proper tab in the chart.	☐	☐	☐
4. Remove guide.	☐	☐	☐
5. Place the folder between the two appropriate existing folders, taking care to place the folder between the two charts.	☐	☐	☐
6. Scan color coding to ensure none of the charts in that section are out of order.	☐	☐	☐
7. AFF Explain what you would do when you find a chart out of order. Should you bring it to the attention of your supervisor?	☐	☐	☐

____

____

____

____

CALCULATION

Total Possible Points: ______

Total Points Earned: ______ Multiplied by 100 = ______ Divided by Total Possible Points = ______ %

PASS ☐ **FAIL** ☐ **COMMENTS:**

Student's signature ______________________ Date ______

Partner's signature ______________________ Date ______

Instructor's signature ______________________ Date ______

CHAPTER 9

Electronic Applications in the Medical Office

Learning Outcomes

Cognitive Domain

1. Spell and define the key words
2. Identify the basic computer components
3. Discuss the importance of routine maintenance of office equipment
4. Explain the basics of connecting to the Internet
5. Discuss the safety concerns for online searching
6. Describe how to use a search engine
7. List sites that can be used by professionals and sites geared for patients
8. Describe the benefits of an intranet and explain how it differs from the Internet
9. Describe the various types of clinical software that might be used in a physician's office
10. Describe the various types of administrative software that might be used in a physician's office
11. Discuss applications of electronic technology in effective communication
12. Describe the considerations for purchasing a computer
13. Describe various training options
14. Discuss the adoption of electronic health records
15. Describe the steps in making the transition from paper to electronic records
16. Discuss the ethics related to computer access

Affective Domain

1. Apply ethical behaviors, including honest/integrity in the performance of medical assisting practice

Psychomotor Domain

1. Care for and maintain computer hardware (Procedure 9-1)
2. Use the Internet to access information related to the medical office (Procedure 9-2)
3. Use office hardware and software to maintain office systems
4. Execute data management using electronic health care records such as the EMR
5. Use office hardware and software to maintain office systems

ABHES Competencies

1. Apply electronic technology
2. Receive, organize, prioritize, and transmit information expediently
3. Locate information and resources for patients and employers
4. Apply computer application skills using variety of different electronic programs including both practice management software and EMR software

Name: ______________________ Date: __________ Grade: __________

COG MULTIPLE CHOICE

1. Another name for a central processing unit is a:
   - a. silicon chip.
   - b. USB port.
   - c. modem.
   - d. microprocessor.
   - e. handheld computer.

2. The purpose of a zip drive in a computer is to:
   - a. scan information.
   - b. delete information.
   - c. store information.
   - d. research information.
   - e. translate information.

3. The acronym *DSL* stands for:
   - a. data storage location.
   - b. digital subscriber line.
   - c. digital storage link.
   - d. data saved/lost.
   - e. digital software link.

4. In a physician's practice, the HIPAA officer:
   - a. checks for security threats or gaps in electronic information.
   - b. purchases new technological equipment.
   - c. maintains computer equipment and fixes problems.
   - d. trains staff in how to use computer equipment.
   - e. monitors staff who may be misusing computer equipment.

Scenario for questions 5 and 6: A parent approaches you and asks how he can keep his 9-year-old daughter safe on the Internet.

5. Which of these actions would you recommend to the parent?
   - a. Don't allow the daughter on the Internet after 7 p.m.
   - b. Stand behind the daughter the entire time she is using the Internet.
   - c. Don't permit the daughter to use the Internet until she is 10 years old.
   - d. Add a filter to the daughter's computer to only allow safe sites as decided by the parent.
   - e. Ask other parents for advice.

6. Which of these Web sites might be helpful to the parent?
   - a. www.skyscape.com
   - b. www.pdacortec.com
   - c. www.ezclaim.com
   - d. www.cyberpatrol.com
   - e. www.nextgen.com

7. To protect your computer from a virus, you should:
   - a. make sure that your computer is correctly shut down every time you use it.
   - b. avoid opening any attachments from unknown Web sites.
   - c. only download material from government Web sites.
   - d. consult a computer technician before you use new software.
   - e. only open one Web site at a time.

8. What is the advantage of encrypting an e-mail?
   - a. It makes the e-mail arrive at its intended destination faster.
   - b. It marks the e-mail as *urgent.*
   - c. It scrambles the e-mail so that it cannot be read until it reaches the recipient.
   - d. It translates the e-mail into another language.
   - e. It informs the sender when the e-mail has been read by the recipient.

9. Which of these is an example of an inappropriate e-mail?

a. "There will be a staff meeting on Wednesday at 9 a.m."

b. "Please return Mrs. Jay's call: Her number is 608-223-3444."

c. "If anyone has seen a lost pair of sunglasses, please return them to reception."

d. "Mr. Orkley thinks he is having a stroke. Please advise."

e. "Mrs. Jones called to confirm her appointment."

10. Which of the following is a peripheral?

a. Zip drive

b. Monitor

c. Keyboard

d. Internet

e. Modem

11. Which of these would you most likely find on an intranet?

a. Advice about health insurance

b. Minutes from staff meetings

c. Information about Medicare

d. Descriptions of alternative treatments

e. National guidelines on medical ethics

12. What is the difference between clinical and administrative software packages?

a. Clinical software helps provide good medical care, whereas administrative software keeps the office efficient.

b. Administrative software is designed to be used by medical assistants, whereas clinical software is used by physicians.

c. Clinical software is cheaper than administrative software because it offers fewer technical features.

d. Administrative software lasts longer than clinical software because it is of higher quality.

e. Clinical software does not allow users to access it without a password, whereas anyone can use administrative software.

13. Which of these should you remember to do when paging a physician?

a. Follow up the page with a phone call to make sure the physician got the message.

b. Keep track of what time the message is sent and repage if there is no response.

c. Document the fact that you sent a page to the physician.

d. Contact the person who left the message to let him or her know you have paged the physician.

e. E-mail the physician with a copy of the paged message.

14. You can use the Meeting Maker software program to:

a. contact patients about appointment changes.

b. coordinate internal meetings and calendars.

c. print patient reminders for annual checkups.

d. create slideshow presentations for meetings.

e. page office staff when a meeting is about to start.

15. Which of these is an important consideration when purchasing a new computer for the office?

a. Whether the computer's programs are HIPAA compliant

b. Whether the computer will be delivered to the office

c. The number of people who will be using the computer

d. The amount of space the computer will take up in the office

e. Which is the best-selling computer on the market

16. When assigning computer log-in passwords to staff, a physician should:

a. make sure that everyone has the code for the hospital computers.

b. give staff two log-in passwords: one for professional use and one for personal use.

c. issue all new employees their own password.

d. make sure that everyone has access to his or her e-mails, in case he or she is out of the office.

e. use a standard log-in password for all the office computers.

17. It is a good idea to lock the hard drive when you are moving a computer to:

   a. prevent the zip drive from falling out.
   b. make sure that no information is erased.
   c. stop viruses from attacking the computer.
   d. protect the CPU and disk drives.
   e. avoid damaging the keyboard.

18. A modem is a(n):

   a. communication device that connects a computer to other computers, including the Internet.
   b. piece of software that enables the user to perform advanced administrative functions.
   c. name for the Internet.
   d. method of storing data on the computer.
   e. type of networking technology for local area networks.

19. Which of the following is true of an abstract found during a literary search?

   a. Abstracts are only found on government Web sites.
   b. Only physicians can access an abstract during a literary search.
   c. An abstract is a summary of a journal article.
   d. Most medical offices cannot afford to download an abstract.
   e. Abstracts can only be printed at a hospital library.

20. If a computer is exposed to static electricity, there is the potential risk of:

   a. electrical fire.
   b. memory loss.
   c. dust accumulation.
   d. slow Internet connection.
   e. viruses.

21. You have been asked to train new employees on how to use an administrative application. However, you do not have a lot of time or extra funding to spend on training. Circle the best option for training the new employees.

   a. Have them read the user manual.
   b. Have them call the help desk.
   c. Have them ask another colleague.
   d. Have them take a tutorial on the program.
   e. Hire experts from the software company.

22. When shopping for prescription management software, what is the minimum that a physician should be able to do with the program? Circle the correct answer.

   a. Find a patient name in a database, write the prescription, and download it to the pharmacy.
   b. Find a patient name in a database, check the prescription for contraindication, and download it to the pharmacy.
   c. Find a patient name in a database, write the prescription, and print it out for the patient.
   d. Find a medication in a database, write the prescription, and download the data to a handheld computer.
   e. Find a patient name in a database, write the prescription, download it to the pharmacy, and check that the medication is covered by insurance.

COG MATCHING

Grade: _____

Match the following key terms to their definitions.

Key Terms

23. _____ cookies
24. _____ downloading
25. _____ encryption
26. _____ Ethernet
27. _____ Internet
28. _____ intranet
29. _____ literary search
30. _____ search engine
31. _____ surfing
32. _____ virus
33. _____ virtual

Definitions

a. a system that allows the computer to be connected to a cable or DSL system
b. a private network of computers that share data
c. a global system used to connect one computer to another
d. tiny files left on your computer's hard drive by a Web site without your permission
e. a dangerous invader that enters your computer through a source and can destroy your files, software programs, and possibly even the hard drive
f. transferring information from an outside location to your computer's hard drive
g. the process of scrambling e-mail messages so that they cannot be read until they reach the recipient
h. the process of navigating Web sites
i. a program that allows you to find information on the Web related to specific terms
j. a search that involves finding journal articles that present new facts or data about a given topic
k. simulated by your computer

COG SHORT ANSWER

Grade: _____

34. List three benefits of having appointment scheduling software in the office.

_____

_____

_____

_____

35. You receive an e-mail from a patient saying that his medication is working out well and is not causing any side effects. He will be in for his appointment next Tuesday. How do you document this information in the patient's medical record?

36. What are three benefits of using electronic health records instead of manual charts?

37. Mr. Jones requires special treatment that uses a laser machine. He makes an appointment for Thursday morning and takes time off work to attend. When he arrives at the facility, he is told that the machine is only available on Mondays and that the new receptionist was unaware of this fact when she made his appointment. How could an administrative software program have helped to prevent this situation?

COG PSY PATIENT EDUCATION Grade: ______

38. A patient has told you of his decision to start buying prescription medication on the Internet. What warnings/information should you give to him?

COG PSY ACTIVE LEARNING

Grade: _______

39. Perform research using the Internet to find information about a disease and possible treatments. Try using different key words to see which ones produce the most useful results. Make a list of the Web sites you have used and observe whether each one has the logo of a verification program such as the HON (Health on the Net) seal.

40. Use the PowerPoint program on the computer to turn your Internet research about a common disease into a presentation. Use the program to make handouts of your presentation for quick office reference. You can use the tutorial feature on the software if you are unsure how to perform certain functions.

41. Visit the Medicare Web site at www.medicare.gov. Find the part of the Web site that addresses FAQs, or frequently asked questions. Choose five of these questions that might be relevant to your patients and print the questions and answers. Then use presentation software to highlight these five questions in a presentation that you will give to your class.

COG IDENTIFICATION

Grade: _______

42. Your office has started converting many of your paper files into digital online files to save time. Recently, you have realized that accessing these records through your Internet service provider (ISP) is taking a very long time. Circle the solutions to this problem.

a. Upgrade your office's ISP to cable.Q2

b. Switch your Web browser.

c. Switch your search engine.

d. Upgrade your printer.

e. Eliminate viruses with a virus scan.

f. Upgrade your monitor.

g. Upgrade your office's ISP to DSL.

43. A patient has asked you for information on how she can lower her cholesterol. You have decided to surf the Internet to find the latest information. Place a check in the "Yes" column for those key words that would lead to a faster, more efficient search. Place a check in the "No" column for those key words that would lead to a slower, less efficient search.

Key Words	Yes	No
a. cholesterol		
b. lowering cholesterol		
c. cholesterol diet		
d. How do people lower their cholesterol?		
e. cholesterol reduction		

44. A diabetic patient has been researching information on the disease. He has asked you to review a list of Web sites he has been reading. Place a check in the "Patient" box for sites that are more useful for patients. Place a check in the "Professional" box for sites that are more useful to physicians and medical assistants.

Web sites	Patient	Professional
a. www.mywebmd.com		
b. www.lancet.org		
c. www.jama.com		
d. www.healthfinder.gov		
e. www.tifaq.com		

COG PSY PATIENT EDUCATION

Grade: ________

45. A patient has expressed an interest in learning more about her food allergies on the Internet. You decide to give her advice on what to look out for when surfing. Place a check in the "Yes" column indicating that the statement is good advice. Place a check in the "No" column indicating that the statement is bad advice.

Key Words	Yes	No
a. Almost all testimonials can be trusted.		
b. Don't trust sites that claim to have secret formulas, medical miracles, or breakthroughs.		
c. Some treatments found online are best to not tell your physician about.		
d. No matter how professional the Web site, you cannot learn lifesaving skills on the Internet.		

TRUE OR FALSE?

Grade: ________

46. Determine whether the following statements are true or false. If false, explain why.

a. The advanced search feature of a search engine should return more results.

____

b. Internal job postings are often found on the Internet.

____

c. The most popular program used to write presentations is PowerPoint.

____

d. A computer system is divided into three areas: hardware, peripherals, and software.

____

AFF PSY WHAT WOULD YOU DO?

Grade: ________

47. You perform most of the administrative tasks in a physician's office, and have been asked for your input concerning a new office computer. The physician asks you which administrative features you would find helpful in a new computer. List three administrative software programs that you would find useful and explain what functions they perform.

____

____

____

____

48. A patient tells you that her medicine has not been working properly and that she is thinking of researching alternative treatments on the Internet. What is the best advice you can give her?

____

____

____

____

49. One of your coworkers has a habit of getting up from her computer and leaving confidential patient information visible on the screen. She says that she sits too far away from patients for them to read anything on the screen, but you have seen several patients near the computer while your coworker is away from her desk. What do you say to her?

____

____

____

____

50. It is your first week working at a physician's office. You notice that the computer is dusty and in the morning sunlight. Disks are in a neat pile next to the uncovered computer. What steps would you take to maintain this computer?

____

____

____

____

AFF CASE STUDY FOR CRITICAL THINKING

Grade: ________

You are teaching a new employee to use the computer system in the office where you work. Ginger is excited and enthusiastic about her new job. At every possible opportunity, Ginger checks her Facebook and Twitter pages. You know that this is against the office policy regarding accepted use of office computers.

51. Circle all appropriate actions from the list below.

- **a.** Beg the office manager to get someone else to train Ginger.
- **b.** Show her the policy in the office *Policies and Procedures Manual.*
- **c.** Tell her if she continues this practice she will get fired.
- **d.** Tell her that the IT department can and will track her use of the office computer.
- **e.** Suggest that she wait until she gets off work for personal computer use.
- **f.** Suggest that people should talk to each other the way they used to, face to face.

52. Circle the accurate statements from the list below. Businesses control personal use of their computers because:

- **a.** it reduces wear and tear on the computers.
- **b.** it is inefficient for employees to be doing personal things while at work.
- **c.** it is dishonest to use someone else's computer.
- **d.** it is unprofessional and unethical.
- **e.** you should never disobey the office rules, no matter what.
- **f.** they are not paying you to be on Facebook and Twitter.
- **g.** it is illegal.

53. You are teaching Ginger how to care for her computer. Why is it important to perform routine maintenance on the office computer? Circle all appropriate answers from the list below.

- **a.** It enhances the performance and prolongs the life of the equipment.
- **b.** It is a rule and you *always* follow the rules, no matter what.
- **c.** It shows that you are a clean person.
- **d.** It looks bad for the patients to see dust.
- **e.** It is in the office *Policy and Procedure Manual.*

PSY **PROCEDURE 9-1** **Care for and Maintain Computer Hardware**

Name: ______________ Date: ________ Time: ________ Grade: ________

EQUIPMENT/SUPPLIES: Computer CPU, monitor, keyboard, mouse, printer, duster, simulated warranties

STANDARDS: Given the needed equipment and a place to work the student will perform this skill with ______% accuracy in a total of ______ minutes. *(Your instructor will tell you what the percentage and time limits will be before you begin.)*

KEY: 4 = Satisfactory 0 = Unsatisfactory NA = this step is not counted

PROCEDURE STEPS	SELF	PARTNER	INSTRUCTOR
1. Place the monitor, keyboard, and printer in a cool, dry area out of direct sunlight.	☐	☐	☐
2. Place the computer desk on an antistatic floor mat or carpet.	☐	☐	☐
3. Clean the monitor screen with antistatic wipes.	☐	☐	☐
4. Use dust covers for the keyboard and the monitor when they are not in use.	☐	☐	☐
5. Lock the hard drive when moving the computer.	☐	☐	☐
6. Keep keyboard and mouse free of debris and liquids; dust and/or vacuum the keyboard.	☐	☐	☐
7. Create a file for maintenance and warranty contracts for the computer system.	☐	☐	☐
8. Handle data storage disks with special care.	☐	☐	☐
9. AFF If you were the office manager, explain how you would respond to an employee who continued to spill soft drinks on her keyboard.	☐	☐	☐

____

____

____

____

CALCULATION

Total Possible Points: ________

Total Points Earned: ________ Multiplied by 100 = ________ Divided by Total Possible Points = ________ %

PASS ☐ **FAIL** ☐ **COMMENTS:**

Student's signature ______________________ Date ______

Partner's signature ______________________ Date ______

Instructor's signature ______________________ Date ______

PSY PROCEDURE 9-2 Searching on the Internet

Name: ______________________ Date: __________ Time: __________ Grade: __________

EQUIPMENT/SUPPLIES: Computer with Web browser software, modem, active Internet connection account

STANDARDS: Given the needed equipment and a place to work the student will perform this skill with _______% accuracy in a total of _______ minutes. *(Your instructor will tell you what the percentage and time limits will be before you begin.)*

KEY: 4 = Satisfactory 0 = Unsatisfactory NA = this step is not counted

PROCEDURE STEPS	SELF	PARTNER	INSTRUCTOR
1. Connect computer to the Internet.	☐	☐	☐
2. Locate a search engine.	☐	☐	☐
3. Select two or three key words and type them at the appropriate place on the Web page.	☐	☐	☐
4. View the number of search results. If no sites are found, check spelling and retype or choose new key words.	☐	☐	☐
5. If the search produces a long list, do an advanced search and refine key words.	☐	☐	☐
6. Select an appropriate site and open its home page.	☐	☐	☐
7. If satisfied with the site's information, either download the material or bookmark the page. If unsatisfied with its information, either visit a site listed on the results page or return to the search engine.	☐	☐	☐
8. AFF You sit down to use your office computer to search for information with a patient when a coworker's Facebook page pops up. You are embarrassed at the unprofessionalism this displays in front of the patient. Explain how you would respond in this situation.	☐	☐	☐

____

____

____

____

CALCULATION

Total Possible Points: ______

Total Points Earned: ______ Multiplied by 100 = ______ Divided by Total Possible Points = ______ %

PASS **FAIL** **COMMENTS:**

☐ ☐

Student's signature ______________________ Date ______

Partner's signature ______________________ Date ______

Instructor's signature ______________________ Date ______

CHAPTER 10

Medical Office Management, Safety, and Emergency Preparedness

Learning Outcomes

Cognitive Domain

1. Spell and define the key terms
2. Describe what is meant by organizational structure
3. List seven responsibilities of the medical office manager
4. Explain the five staffing issues that a medical office manager will be responsible for handling
5. List the types of policies and procedures that should be included in a medical office's policy and procedures manual
6. List five types of promotional materials that a medical office may distribute
7. Discuss financial concerns that the medical office manager must be capable of addressing
8. Describe the duties regarding office maintenance, inventory, and service contracts
9. Discuss the need for continuing education
10. Describe liability, professional, personal injury and third-party insurance
11. List three services provided by most medical malpractice companies
12. List six guidelines for completing incident reports
13. List four regulatory agencies that require medical offices to have quality improvement programs
14. Describe the accreditation process of The Joint Commission
15. Describe the steps to developing a quality improvement program
16. Identify safety techniques that can be used to prevent accidents and maintain a safe work environment
17. Describe the importance of Material Safety Data Sheets (MSDS) in a health care setting
18. Identify safety signs, symbols, and labels
19. Describe fundamental principles for evacuation of a health care setting
20. Discuss fire safety issues in a health care environment
21. Discuss requirements for responding to hazardous material disposal
22. Identify principles of body mechanics and ergonomics
23. Discuss critical elements of an emergency plan for response to a natural disaster or other emergency
24. Identify emergency preparedness plans in your community
25. Discuss potential role(s) of the medical assistant in emergency preparedness
26. List and discuss legal and illegal interview questions
27. Discuss all levels of governmental legislation and regulation as they apply to medical assisting practice, including FDA and DEA regulations
28. Apply local, state and federal health care legislation and regulation appropriate to the medical assisting practice setting
29. Describe basic elements of first aid
30. Identify how the Americans with Disabilities Act (ADA) applies to the medical assisting profession

Psychomotor Domain

1. Create a policy and procedures manual (Procedure 10-1)
2. Perform an office inventory (Procedure 10-2)
3. Perform within scope of practice
4. Select appropriate barrier/personal protective equipment (PPE) for potentially infectious situations
5. Assist physician with patient care

6. Report relevant information to others succinctly and accurately
7. Evaluate the work environment to identify safe versus unsafe working conditions
8. Maintain a current list of community resources for emergency preparedness
9. Develop a personal (patient and employee) safety plan
10. Develop an environmental safety plan
11. Demonstrate proper use of the following equipment: eyewash, fire extinguishers, sharps disposal containers
12. Participate in a mock environmental exposure with documentation of steps taken
13. Explain the evacution plan for a physician's office
14. Demonstrate methods of fire prevention in the health care setting
15. Complete an incident report
16. Incorporate the Patient's Bill of Rights into personal practice and medical office policies and procedures
17. Apply local, state and federal health care legislation and regulation appropriate to the medical assisting practice setting

Affective Domain

1. Recognize the effects of stress on all persons involved in emergency situations
2. Demonstrate self-awareness in responding to emergency situations
3. Apply active listening skills
4. Use appropriate body language and other nonverbal skills in communicating with patients, family, and staff
5. Recognize the importance of local, state and federal legislation and regulation in the practice setting

ABHES Competencies

1. Perform routine maintenance of administrative and clinical equipment
2. Maintain inventory, equipment and supplies
3. Maintain medical facility
4. Serve as liaison between physician and others
5. Interview effectively
6. Comprehend the current employment outlook for the medical assistant
7. Understand the importance of maintaining liability coverage once employed in the industry
8. Perform risk management procedures
9. Comply with federal, state and local health laws and regulations

Name: ______________________ Date: __________ Grade: __________

COG MULTIPLE CHOICE

Scenario for questions 1 and 2: It's your first day on the job as the medical office manager, so there's a lot you don't know yet about this office.

1. You want to know who's responsible for what in the office. Where is the best place to find that information?
   - **a.** Payroll records
   - **b.** The work schedule
   - **c.** The chain-of-command chart
   - **d.** The recent employee evaluations
   - **e.** The bulletin board

2. You know the office is running low on paper and syringes. You're most likely to find out how to order supplies in:
   - **a.** the QI plan.
   - **b.** the service contracts folder.
   - **c.** the operating budget.
   - **d.** the policy and procedures manual.
   - **e.** the communication notebook.

3. An MSDS is required to contain:
   - **a.** general information about safety.
   - **b.** a written hazard communication plan.
   - **c.** information regarding hazardous chemicals found in a facility.
   - **d.** the appropriate amount of bleach that can be stored in a medical office.
   - **e.** a complete list of the hazardous materials in a facility.

4. The office keeps running out of tongue depressors. Which action should you take first?
   - **a.** Establish a recycling program.
   - **b.** Determine whether someone is stealing supplies.
   - **c.** Review the system for keeping track of supplies.
   - **d.** Tell the physicians not to use so many tongue depressors.
   - **e.** Borrow some tongue depressors from the nearest medical office.

5. Which item should be in any job description?
   - **a.** Age requirements
   - **b.** Salary or hourly pay
   - **c.** Physical requirements
   - **d.** The preferred gender of the applicant
   - **e.** Medical and dental benefits

6. Which task should you be expected to perform as medical office manager?
   - **a.** Clean the waiting room
   - **b.** Assign someone to make coffee
   - **c.** Develop promotional pamphlets
   - **d.** Assist with simple medical procedures
   - **e.** Sign prescription refills

7. Which of the following is a medical office manager's responsibility?
   - **a.** Completing all incident reports
   - **b.** Teaching CPR
   - **c.** Evaluating the physicians
   - **d.** Hiring and firing employees
   - **e.** Teaching employees about malpractice insurance

8. Which statement is true of an incident report about a patient?
   - **a.** It should be mailed to the attorney of your choice.
   - **b.** It should be written by a physician.
   - **c.** It should be written within 24 hours of the incident.
   - **d.** It should be written from the patient's point of view.
   - **e.** It should be kept in the medical office.

9. Which action should be taken if an employee is stuck by a patient's needle?

   a. The patient should be informed.
   b. The physician should take disciplinary action against the employee.
   c. The employee should write an incident report.
   d. The employee should be kept away from patients.
   e. The employee should sign a form admitting liability.

10. Which of the following categories is part of a capital budget?

   a. Payroll
   b. Medical supplies
   c. Building maintenance
   d. Heating and air conditioning
   e. Electricity

11. Which item should be part of any medical office budget?

   a. Merit bonuses
   b. Billing service
   c. Continuing education
   d. Magazine subscriptions
   e. Children's play facility

12. Which agency licenses and monitors health care organizations and enforces regulations?

   a. CMS
   b. State health department
   c. The Joint Commission
   d. OSHA
   e. HCFA

13. General liability and medical malpractice insurance is for:

   a. all medical professionals.
   b. all physicians.
   c. physicians who perform risky procedures.
   d. medical professionals with high risk profiles.
   e. physicians and nurses.

14. The first step in creating a quality improvement plan is to:

   a. form a task force.
   b. identify the problem.
   c. establish a monitoring plan.
   d. assign an expected threshold.
   e. explore the problem.

15. Which of the following items should be included in an emergency kit?

   a. Alcohol wipes
   b. Syringe
   c. Penicillin
   d. Oscilloscope
   e. Sample containers

16. If you fill out an incident report, you should:

   a. keep a copy of the report.
   b. have a supervisor review it.
   c. give your title but not your name.
   d. fill out only the sections that apply.
   e. summarize what happened in the report.

17. The 2001 discovery of anthrax in an envelope to be delivered to a U.S. Congressman is an example of a(n):

   a. bioterrorist attack.
   b. epidemic.
   c. pandemic.
   d. ergonomics.
   e. ADF.

18. Which of the following is used to estimate expenditures and revenues?

   a. Budget
   b. Tracking file
   c. Expected threshold
   d. Financial statement
   e. Previous expenditures

19. Risk management is a(n):

a. process begun only after a sentinel event.

b. process intended to identify potential problems.

c. external process that deals with OSHA violations.

d. internal process that deals with recurring problems.

e. process undertaken by managers to reduce annual expenditure.

20. Which of the following is true of an expected threshold for a quality improvement program?

a. It is the expected percentage reduction in risk.

b. It is a way to measure the success of the program.

c. It should be set higher for more dangerous problems.

d. It should be set lower than you think you can achieve.

e. It should only be used for particularly severe problems.

21. General liability and medical malpractice insurance is needed:

a. only by employees in offices that use new medical procedures.

b. by physicians sued for malpractice, but not by nurses or office personnel.

c. to protect medical professionals from financial loss due to lawsuits or settlements.

d. because visitors who are hurt in the waiting room can sue unless an incident report is completed.

COG MATCHING

Grade: ______

Match the following key terms to their definitions.

Key Terms	Definitions
22. _____ bioterrorism	**a.** numerical goal for a given problem
23. _____ body mechanics	**b.** statement of work-related responsibilities
24. _____ budget	**c.** series of steps required to perform a given task
25. _____ compliance officer	**d.** written account of untoward patient, visitor, or staff event
26. _____ epidemic	**e.** description of the goals of the practice and whom it serves
27. _____ ergonomics	**f.** statement regarding the organization's rules on a given topic
28. _____ expected threshold	**g.** purposeful infliction of a dangerous agent into a populated area with intent to harm
29. _____ incident report	**h.** financial planning tool used to estimate anticipated expenditures and revenues
30. _____ job description	**i.** staff member who ensures compliance with the rules and regulations of the office
31. _____ mission statement	**j.** implementation of practices that will help ensure high-quality patient care and service
32. _____ organizational chart	**k.** flow sheet that allows staff to identify team members and see where they fit into the team
33. _____ pandemic	**l.** group of employees with different roles brought together to solve a problem
34. _____ policy	**m.** using the correct muscles and posture to complete a task safely and efficiently
35. _____ procedure	**n.** the study of the fit between a worker and his/her physical work environment
36. _____ quality improvement	**o.** a disease affecting many people in a specific geographic area
37. _____ task force	**p.** a disease infecting numerous people in many areas of the world at the same time

SHORT ANSWER

Grade: _______

38. List three responsibilities of the office manager regarding service contractors.

____

____

____

____

39. List five types of promotional materials that a medical office might use.

____

____

____

____

40. List six items that should be included in employee fire safety training.

____

____

____

____

41. List the four basic requirements of the hazard communication standard.

____

____

____

____

42. List the four basic principles of proper body mechanics.

43. List five techniques used to reduce fatigue as you work.

COG IDENTIFICATION

Grade: ________

44. Below is a list of the steps for creating a quality improvement plan. Put the steps in logical order. Then explain the reason for each step.

Steps

Assign an expected threshold.
Document the entire process.
Establish a monitoring plan.
Explore the problem and propose solutions.
Form a task force.
Identify the problem.
Implement the solution.
Obtain feedback.

Step	Reason
1.	
2.	
3.	
4.	
5.	
6.	
7.	
8.	

COG YES OR NO?

Grade: ________

Answer "Yes," "No," or "Yes But" to the following questions about evaluating employees. If you answer "No" or "Yes But," be able to explain why.

	Yes	No	Yes But ...
45. Are employee evaluations your responsibility as a medical office manager?			
46. Should new employees be evaluated annually?			
47. Should you coach new employees about how to do their jobs well?			
48. Can annual performance appraisals be done orally?			
49. Should you communicate with employees about performance problems when one of the physicians asks you to?			
50. Should you inform a good employee yearly that she or he is doing a good job?			

COG IDENTIFICATION

Grade: ________

51. Medical offices usually have an operating budget and a capital budget. Separate the following items into the two categories by checking the column for operating budget or capital budget.

Budget Item	Operating Budget	Capital Budget
a. payroll		
b. medical equipment		
c. office supplies		
d. Internet service		
e. medical supplies		
f. building maintenance		
g. telephone service		
h. electricity		
i. expensive furniture		
j. patient materials		
k. continuing education		

COG PSY ACTIVE LEARNING

Grade: ________

52. When you complete your program of study, you would like to find a job as a medical office manager. Write the job description for your ideal job. Be sure to include all the essential elements, including a position summary, hours, location, and duties.

53. Your office manager has assigned you to a task force that will write a plan for fire prevention in your office. Your role in the group is to establish the headings for the plan. List five items that should be included.

____

____

____

____

54. The task force did such a good job with the last assignment, they are now asked to write the emergency action plan for your office as well. List the six items that should be included.

____

____

____

____

55. Working together with a partner, search the local classified ads for an open job as a medical office manager. Then prepare to role-play the interview process with your partner, taking turns acting as the interviewer and the interviewee. Make a list of questions that you would ask as both the interviewer and the interviewee. Switch places so you both get to experience the job interview process from each perspective.

____

____

____

____

COG IDENTIFICATION

Grade: _______

56. Circle all the following tasks that are the responsibility of the medical office manager.

a. scheduling staff

b. ordering supplies

c. writing the budget

d. keeping up to date on legal issues

e. assisting with medical procedures

f. cleaning the office and waiting room

g. revising policy and procedures manuals

h. presenting continuing education seminars

i. developing HIPAA and OSHA regulations

j. developing promotional pamphlets or newsletters

57. Inventory control is the responsibility of the office manager. On the checklist below, put an **M** beside the inventory tasks the manager should do and an **A** beside the things an assistant or other office staff member can do.

_____ Receive supplies

_____ Initial the packing slip

_____ Develop a system to keep track of supplies

_____ Determine the procedures for ordering supplies

_____ Transfer supplies from packing boxes to supply shelves

_____ Check the packing slip against the actual supply contents

_____ Keep receipts or packing slips in a bills-pending file for payment

_____ Develop a process to check that deliveries of supplies are complete and accurate

COG YES OR NO?

Grade: ________

58. Indicate by a check mark in the "Yes" or "No" column whether an item should be included in a medical office's policy and procedures manual.

Policy	Yes	No
a. a chain-of-command chart		
b. a list of employee benefits		
c. infection control guidelines		
d. the office operating budget		
e. annual employee evaluations		
f. procedures for bill collections		
g. copies of completed incident reports		
h. a description of the goals of the practice		
i. responsibilities and procedures for ordering supplies		
j. a list of responsibilities for the last employee to leave the office each day		

COG LISTING

Grade: ________

59. List six of the elements that should be included in any job description.

a. ____________________

b. ____________________

c. ____________________

d. ____________________

e. ____________________

f. ____________________

60. In addition to writing job descriptions and managing employee evaluations, list the three other staffing issues that are the responsibility of the medical office manager?

a. ____________________

b. ____________________

c. ____________________

61. List three services provided by most medical malpractice companies.

a. ____________________

b. ____________________

c. ____________________

COG FALSE THEN TRUE

Grade: _________

62. Each of the following statements about incident reports is false or incomplete. Rewrite each statement to make it true and complete.

   a. You should write up an incident report as the event was reported to you.

   ____

   b. The witness should summarize and explain the event.

   ____

   c. You should remain anonymous when you fill out a report.

   ____

   d. The form should be completed within 48 hours of the event.

   ____

   e. If a particular section of the report does not apply, it should be left blank.

   ____

   f. Keep a copy of the incident report for your own personal record.

   ____

   g. If the incident happened to a patient, put a copy of the report in the patient's chart.

   ____

   h. The report should be reviewed by a supervisor to make sure the office is not liable.

   ____

   i. Incident reports are written when negative events happen to patients or visitors.

   ____

COG MATCHING

Grade: _________

63. Below is a list of four regulatory agencies that require medical offices to have quality improvement programs. Draw a line between the two columns to match the regulatory agency with its description.

Agencies	Descriptions
1. CMS	a. federal agency that regulates and runs Medicare and Medicaid
2. OSHA	b. nonfederal agency to license and monitor health care organizations and enforce regulations
3. The Joint Commission	c. federal agency that enforces regulations to protect the health and welfare of patients and employees
4. state health department	d. agency that sets voluntary health care standards and evaluates a health care organization's implementation of those standards

COG WHICH IS WHICH?

Grade: ______

64. Explain how quality improvement programs and risk management work together in a medical office.

______

______

______

______

COG TRUE OR FALSE?

Grade: ______

65. Determine whether the following statements are true or false. If false, explain why.

a. Health care organizations are required to follow the regulations of the Joint Commission.

______

b. Accreditation by The Joint Commission is valid for 5 years.

______

c. If The Joint Commission's initial site review identifies unsatisfactory areas, the health care organization may later prove that corrections have been made by passing a focus survey.

______

d. The health care organization should prepare for the Joint Commission survey by assessing its compliance with OSHA standards.

______

AFF WHAT WOULD YOU DO?

Grade: _______

66. As you enter the office on the first day of your new job as the medical office manager, you notice a thick layer of dust on the plastic plants in the waiting room and see that the magazines are old and tattered. The staff greets you with enthusiasm, saying you are just what they need to deal with the patients' complaints about spending too much time waiting to be seen. Someone has left an incident report file on your desk. You look through it right away and learn that a needlestick has been reported almost every Wednesday evening for a month. What would you do first, and why?

67. You have a patient who lost her home and several pets to a recent tornado in your city. You know she is at risk for the development of a major psychiatric disorder. What are five ways to help this patient who has been exposed to trauma from natural or manmade disasters?

68. Mrs. Hadley, who is blind and walks with a cane, slipped on the wet floor near a leaky water cooler and fell, cutting her forearm. One of the nurses examined and treated her wound and apologized. Mrs. Hadley said it was no problem and left the office. The nurse told you she wasn't going to file an incident report because the wound was minor and Mrs. Hadley had accepted her apology. As the medical office manager, what should you do?

AFF CASE STUDY FOR CRITICAL THINKING

Grade: _______

You have been asked by your physician-employer to inspect the office for possible safety hazards. He wants a report of any negative findings by the end of the week.

69. Circle the most appropriate first step.

- **a.** Ask if you can assign a task force to help you.
- **b.** Design a form for checking off items as you inspect them.
- **c.** Tell him you are too busy with patients to take on such a large task.
- **d.** Call the local fire department to perform the inspection.
- **e.** Call the local OSHA representative to perform the inspection.

70. From the following list of actions, circle all that are appropriate.

- **a.** Check closets for the storage of flammable liquids.
- **b.** Check areas where oxygen is in use.
- **c.** Check to be sure all cylinders and tanks that contain flammable gases or liquids are uncapped and ready for use.
- **d.** Check to see that equipment and carts are on the right side of each hallway.
- **e.** Check the CMA schedule to be sure there is enough coverage to keep everyone safe.

PSY PROCEDURE 10-1 Create a Procedures Manual

Name: ______________________ Date: __________ Time: __________ Grade: __________

EQUIPMENT/SUPPLIES: Word processor, three-ring binder, paper, choose any procedure approved by your instructor

STANDARDS: Given the needed equipment and a place to work the student will perform this skill with _______% accuracy in a total of _______ minutes. *(Your instructor will tell you what the percentage and time limits will be before you begin.)*

KEY: 4 = Satisfactory 0 = Unsatisfactory NA = this step is not counted

PROCEDURE STEPS	SELF	PARTNER	INSTRUCTOR
1. Check the latest information from key governmental agencies, local and state health departments, and health care organizations, such as OSHA, CDC, The Joint Commission, etc. to make sure that the policies and procedures being written comply with federal and state legislation and regulations.	☐	☐	☐
2. Gather product information; consult government agencies, if needed. Secure educational pamphlets.	☐	☐	☐
3. Title the procedure properly.	☐	☐	☐
4. Number the procedure appropriately.	☐	☐	☐
5. Define the overall purpose of the procedure in a sentence or two explaining the intent of the procedure.	☐	☐	☐
6. List all necessary equipment and forms. Include everything needed to complete the task.	☐	☐	☐
7. List each step with its rationale.	☐	☐	☐
8. Provide spaces for signatures.	☐	☐	☐
9. Record the date the procedure was written.	☐	☐	☐
10. AFF Describe how you would explain to employees why they were asked to work in a group to create a procedure manual.	☐	☐	☐

____

____

____

____

CALCULATION

Total Possible Points: ______

Total Points Earned: ______ Multiplied by 100 = ______ Divided by Total Possible Points = ______ %

PASS **FAIL** **COMMENTS:**

☐ ☐

Student's signature ______________________ Date ______

Partner's signature ______________________ Date ______

Instructor's signature ______________________ Date ______

PSY PROCEDURE 10-2 Perform an Office Inventory

Name: ______________________ Date: __________ Time: __________ Grade: __________

EQUIPMENT: Inventory form, reorder form

STANDARDS: Given the needed equipment and a place to work the student will perform this skill with ________% accuracy in a total of __________ minutes. *(Your instructor will tell you what the percentage and time limits will be before you begin.)*

KEY: 4 = Satisfactory 0 = Unsatisfactory NA = this step is not counted

PROCEDURE STEPS	SELF	PARTNER	INSTRUCTOR
1. Using forms supplied by your instructor, count and record the amounts of specified supplies	☐	☐	☐
2. Record amount of each item.	☐	☐	☐
3. Compare amount on hand with amount needed.	☐	☐	☐
4. Complete reorder form based on these numbers.	☐	☐	☐
5. Submit reorder forms to office manager.	☐	☐	☐
6. Document your actions per the ordering procedure.	☐	☐	☐
7. AFF Explain how you would respond to an employee who continually takes a vacation day when the office plans to take inventory.	☐	☐	☐

____

____

____

____

CALCULATION

Total Possible Points: ________

Total Points Earned: ________ Multiplied by 100 = ________ Divided by Total Possible Points = ________ %

PASS ☐ **FAIL** ☐ **COMMENTS:**

Student's signature ______________________________ Date ______

Partner's signature ______________________________ Date ______

Instructor's signature ______________________________ Date ______

WORK PRODUCT 1

Grade: ________

USE METHODS OF QUALITY CONTROL

Louise Baggins, a 55-year-old patient, was visiting the physician for a physical exam. While waiting for her appointment, she asked you to direct her to the restroom. On her way into the restroom, she slipped and fell on a magazine that had fallen on the floor in the reception area. You did not see her fall, but she yelled out in pain after she fell. She was able to get up on her own but injured her wrist. Her wrist was immediately red, swollen, and painful to touch. Dr. Mikuski looked at her wrist and suggested she go to the hospital emergency room to have x-rays. You called an ambulance to transfer Mrs. Baggins to the hospital. Fill in the incident report below to document this event.

Workplace Requirements Program for Safety and Health

SUPERVISOR'S ACCIDENT REPORT FORM

This form is to be completed by the supervisor and forwarded to the Payroll Coordinator along with a copy of the North Carolina Industrial Commission Form 19 (Workers Compensation Form) within five days of the accident. All accidents involving serious bodily injury or death must be reported to the safety and health officer immediately.

ACCIDENT DATA

1. NAME OF EMPLOYEE:
or Patient

2. ADDRESS AND PHONE NO:

3. WORK DEPT. OR DIVISION:

4. SEX: ☐ MALE ☐ FEMALE

5. DATE AND TIME OF INJURY:

6. NATURE OF INJURY:

7. PART OF BODY INJURED:

8. CAUSE OF INJURY:

9. LOCATION OF ACCIDENT:

10. OCCUPATION AND ACTIVITY OF PERSON AT TIME OF ACCIDENT:

11. STATUS OF JOB OR ACTIVITY: (CHOOSE ONE)
Halted

12. NAME AND PHONE NO. OF ACCIDENT WITNESS:

13. LIST UNSAFE ACT, IF ANY:

14. LIST UNSAFE PHYSICAL OR MECHANICAL CONDITION, IF ANY:

15. UNSAFE PERSONAL FACTOR:

16. LIST HAZARD CONTROLS IN EFFECT AT TIME OF INJURY DESIGNED TO PREVENT INJURY:

17. PERSONAL PROTECTIVE EQUIPMENT BEING USED AT TIME OF ACCIDENT:
GLOVES, SAFETY GLASSES, GOGGLES, FACE SHIELD, OTHER

18. BRIEF DESCRIPTION OF ACCIDENT:

19. CORRECTIVE ACTION TAKEN OR RECOMMENDED TO DEPARTMENT SAFETY COMMITTEE:

TREATMENT DATA

20. WAS INJURED TAKEN TO (CHOOSE ONE): Hospital

21. DIAGNOSIS AND TREATMENT, IF KNOWN:

22. ESTIMATED LOST WORKDAYS: ________
(EXCLUDING DAY OF ACCIDENT)

23. DATE OF REPORT:

Month	Day	Year

24. REPORT PREPARED BY:

25. SIGNATURE OF SUPERVISOR:

26. SIGNATURE OF AGENCY SAFETY AND HEALTH OFFICER:

WORK PRODUCT 2

Grade: ________

USE METHODS OF QUALITY CONTROL

After Mrs. Baggins fell in the reception area (see Work Product 1), your supervisor asks you to review any other injuries in the reception area in the past 6 months. There are seven incident reports involving patient falls, and all of those occurred in some part of the reception area. Three patients slipped by the doorway on rainy days. Two more tripped on the corner of the doormat. The last two patients fell in the main lobby—one tripped over a children's toy, and the other slipped on a magazine, just like Mrs. Baggins did.

You are named to represent the medical assistants on a task force addressing these complaints. Assign an expected threshold using measurable, realistic goals. Explore the problem and propose solutions. Establish a QI monitoring plan explaining how data will be collected. Document the entire process and print the information to attach to this sheet. Using the blank memorandum below, write a memo to the staff with instructions to implement the solutions.

Memo

To:

From:

Date:

Re:

UNIT THREE

Managing the Finances in the Practice

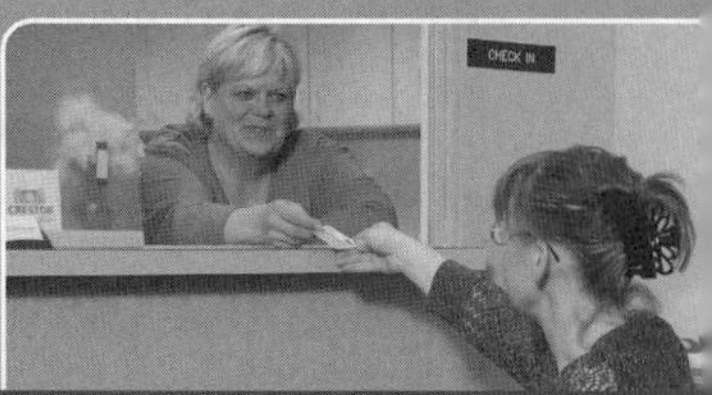

CHAPTER 11

Credit and Collections

Learning Outcomes

Cognitive Domain

1. Spell and define the key terms
2. Discuss physician's fee schedules
3. Discuss forms of payment
4. Explain the legal considerations in extending credit
5. Discuss the legal implications of credit collection
6. Discuss procedures for collecting outstanding accounts
7. Describe the impact of both the Fair Debt Collection Act and the Federal Truth in Lending Act of 1968 as they apply to collections
8. Describe the concept of RBRVS
9. Define Diagnosis-Related Groups (DRGs)
10. Describe the implications of HIPAA for the medical assistant in various medical settings
11. Discuss all levels of government legislation and regulation as they apply to medical assisting practice, including FDA and DEA regulations

Psychomotor Domain

1. Evaluate and manage a patient account (Procedure 11-1)
2. Write a collection letter (Procedure 11-2)
3. Perform collection procedures

Affective Domain

1. Apply ethical behaviors, including honesty and integrity in performance of medical assisting practice
2. Demonstrate sensitivity and professionalism in handling accounts receivable activities with clients
3. Demonstrate sensitivity to patient rights
4. Recognize the importance of local, state, and federal legislation and regulations in the practice setting

ABHES Competencies

1. Perform billing and collection procedures
2. Use physician fee schedule

Name: ______________________ Date: __________ Grade: __________

COG MULTIPLE CHOICE

1. The total of all the charges posted to patients' accounts for the month of May is $16,000. The revenues the practice received for May total $12,000. What is the collection percentage for May?
   a. 5%
   b. 25%
   c. 75%
   d. 80%
   e. 133%

2. Interest that may be charged to a patient account is determined by:
   a. the physician.
   b. the patient.
   c. the insurance company.
   d. the law.
   e. the state.

3. In the UCR concept, the letters stand for:
   a. user, customer, and regulation.
   b. usual, competitive, and regular.
   c. usage, consumption, and return.
   d. usual, customary, and reasonable.
   e. usage, complaint, and rationale.

4. When credit cards are accepted by a medical practice, the medical practice generally agrees to pay the credit card company:
   a. 5.2%.
   b. 1.8%.
   c. 15%.
   d. 3.1%
   e. 25%.

5. Federal regulations require each medical office to describe its services and procedures and to give the procedure codes and prices by:
   a. giving a list to each patient at check in.
   b. offering the list to each patient at payment.
   c. posting a sign stating that a list is available.
   d. answering a patient's questions about billing.
   e. placing an ad in the newspaper describing the fees.

6. Physicians who chose to become participating providers with third-party payers usually do so in order to:
   a. charge higher fees.
   b. simplify fee schedules.
   c. build a solid patient base.
   d. reduce the time before payment.
   e. share a patient load with another physician.

7. It is a good and ethical business practice to:
   a. take payment in cash only.
   b. accept only patients who have insurance.
   c. refuse patients who have third-party payment plans.
   d. discuss fees with patients before they see a physician or nurse.
   e. charge the patient a small fee for paying with a credit card.

8. When dealing with a new patient, you should avoid:
   a. taking cash.
   b. taking a partial payment.
   c. taking a check with two picture IDs.
   d. taking co-payment with an insurance card.
   e. taking a payment by credit card.

9. Most fees for medical services:

a. are paid by insurance companies.

b. are paid by Medicare and Medicaid.

c. are paid by patients who are private payers.

d. are written off on the practice's federal taxes.

e. are paid to the physician late.

10. When an insurance adjustment is made to a fee:

a. the patient is charged less than the normal rate.

b. the medical office receives more than its normal rate.

c. the insurance carrier pays the adjustment rate.

d. the insurance carrier's explanation of benefits shows how much the office may collect for the service.

e. the difference between the physician's normal fee and the insurance carrier's allowed fee is written off.

11. Why would a medical office extend credit to a patient?

a. To save money

b. To accommodate the patient

c. To postpone paying income tax

d. To charge interest

e. To make billing more cost effective

12. Why do many medical offices outsource their credit and billing functions?

a. They don't want to ask their patients for money directly.

b. They are not licensed to manage credit card transactions.

c. Creating their own installment plans is too complicated legally.

d. Managing patient accounts themselves costs about $5 per month per patient.

e. Billing companies can manage the accounts more cost effectively.

13. It is illegal for a medical office to:

a. use a collection agency.

b. disclose fee information to patients who have insurance.

c. deny credit to patients because they receive public assistance.

d. charge patients interest, finance charges, or late fees on unpaid balances.

e. change their established billing cycle

14. If you are attempting to collect a debt from a patient, you must:

a. use reasonable self-restraint.

b. call the patient only at home.

c. hire a licensed bill collection agency.

d. first take the patient to small claims court.

e. wait one year before you can ask for payment.

15. When first attempting to collect a debt by telephone, you should:

a. ask the patient to come in for a checkup.

b. contact the patient before 8:00 a.m. or after 9:00 p.m.

c. contact the patient only at his place of employment.

d. leave a message explaining the situation on the answering machine.

e. speak only to the patient or leave only your first name and number.

16. When you are collecting a debt from an estate, it is best to:

a. send a final bill to the estate's executor.

b. take the matter directly to small claims court.

c. try to collect within a week of the patient's death.

d. allow the family a month to mourn before asking for payment.

e. ask a collection agency to contact the family.

17. If a billing cycle is to be changed, you are legally required to notify patients:

a. 1 month before their payment is due.

b. before the next scheduled appointment.

c. 3 months prior to the billing change.

d. after you approve the change with the insurance company.

e. only if they have outstanding payments.

18. When you age an account, you:

a. write off debts that have been outstanding longer than 120 days.

b. send bills first to the patients who had the most recent procedures.

c. organize patient accounts by how long they have been seeing the physician.

d. calculate the time between the last bill and the date of the last payment.

e. determine the time between the procedure and the date of the last payment.

19. A cancellation of an unpaid debt is called a(n):

a. professional courtesy.

b. co-payment.

c. write-off.

d. adjustment.

e. credit.

20. Which collections method takes the least staff time?

a. Using a collection agency

b. Going to small claims court

c. Billing the patient monthly until paid

d. Scheduling all payments on the first of the month

e. Reporting patients to the credit bureaus

COG MATCHING

Grade: _________

Match the following key terms to their definitions.

Key Terms	Definitions
21. _____ adjustment	**a.** change in a posted account
22. _____ aging schedule	**b.** balance in one's favor on an account.
23. _____ collections	**c.** process of seeking payment for overdue bills
24. _____ credit	**d.** arrangement for a patient to pay on an installment plan
25. _____ installment	**e.** charging other health care professionals a reduced rate
26. _____ participating provider	**f.** cancellation of an unpaid debt.
27. _____ patient co-payment	**g.** a certain share of the bill that a managed care company usually requires the patient to pay
28. _____ professional courtesy	**h.** physician who agrees to participate with managed care companies and other third-party payers
29. _____ write-off	**i.** record of a patient's name, balance, payments made, time of outstanding debt, and relevant comments

COG SHORT ANSWER

Grade: ________

30. Fee setting also considers RBRVS, by which fees are adjusted for geographical differences. What does RBRVS stand for?

31. There should be a sign posted in the office, where patients can see it, giving information about procedure fees. What should be on the sign?

32. Which third-party payers affect fee schedules if the physicians in your office are participating providers, and how many fee schedules might there be?

33. How many times should you contact patients asking them to pay overdue bills? Why?

34. How often should you ask the patient for his or her insurance card, and what should you do with it when you get it?

____

____

____

____

35. What are the three most common ways of collecting overdue accounts?

____

____

____

____

36. What are some of the negative aspects of extending credit to patients? Consider costs, patient attitudes, and legal requirements in your answer.

____

____

____

____

COG ACTIVE LEARNING

Grade: ________

37. Use the Internet to research the three major credit bureaus and find out how to check a new patient's credit history. Specifically, find out what's available to help you decide how to handle payment from people without traditional credit histories. This group includes college students, young adults, recent immigrants, traditional housewives, and people who choose not to use credit cards.

38. Many people feel uncomfortable asking other people for money. However, you need to feel comfortable discussing finance and account information with patients. Working with a partner, role-play a scenario in which a patient has an overdue account that the medical assistant must address. Take turns playing the parts of the medical assistant and the patient to understand both perspectives.

39. In recent years, the government has called into question the practice of professional courtesy extended to other health care professionals. Perform research online or talk to health care professionals to find out more about the issues surrounding professional courtesy. Then write a viewpoint paper arguing for or against the practice of professional courtesy.

COG FALSE THEN TRUE

Grade: _______

40. All the statements below are false or inaccurate. Rewrite each statement so that it accurately reflects the consumer protection laws regarding credit collection.

a. You cannot contact a patient directly about an unpaid bill.

____

b. You should not try to contact a debtor before 9:00 a.m. or after 5:00 p.m.

____

c. You have every right to call debtors at work.

____

d. You should keep calling a patient about a debt after turning the case over to a collection agency, in order to increase your chances of recovering the money.

____

e. It's okay to use abusive language to intimidate a debtor, as long as you don't give false or misleading information.

____

f. If a patient dies and the estate can't meet all of his or her debts, the probate court will pay the medical bills first.

____

COG SHORT ANSWER

Grade: _______

41. List three situations in which calling a patient to collect an overdue payment may be least helpful.

____

____

____

____

42. What should be in a mailing that asks a patient to settle an overdue account?

____

____

____

____

43. What is a good way to use a patient's visit as an opportunity to try to collect payment on an overdue bill?

____

____

____

____

44. What should you say and not say if you call a patient to collect on a bill and you are asked to leave a message?

____

____

____

____

COG TRUE OR FALSE?

Grade: ________

45. Determine whether the following statements are true or false. If false, explain why.

a. A physician's fee schedule takes into consideration the costs of operating the office, such as rent, utilities, malpractice insurance, and salaries.

____

b. If a patient has insurance, you must charge him the insurance carrier's allowed fee for a procedure.

____

c. To maintain good relations with patients, you should be vague and polite when you ask them to pay their bills.

____

d. You should monitor the activity on a patient's credit account in order to keep the collection ratio low.

____

PSY AFF WHAT WOULD YOU DO?

Grade: ________

46. You have several patients who have long-standing debts. They don't come into the office anymore, and they don't respond to your telephone calls or letters. You outsourced your overdue billing to a collections agency but these longtime patients have told you that they have been very upset by the "nastiness" of the collections people who contacted them.

You spoke with a collections agency representative who assured you his employees were doing nothing illegal or inappropriate. You have considered changing collection agencies; but this one's rates are better, and they did collect the debts. What would you do?

____

____

____

____

47. Mrs. Sanchez is seeing Dr. Roland for the first time and has asked you to explain the physician's fees. How would you explain to Mrs. Sanchez how Dr. Roland establishes the fees he charges his patients?

____

____

____

____

AFF CASE STUDY FOR CRITICAL THINKING

Grade: ________

Mr. Green has been a patient with your practice for more than 20 years and has always paid his co-payment or bill before he left the office. Recently, however, he has not been paying anything at all, and his outstanding bill is 60 days past due. You have called his home and left several phone messages, but you still haven't heard from him.

48. What should you do? Circle all appropriate actions from the following list.

a. Send him a letter demanding that he pay his balance immediately.

b. Flag his account for the credit manager to speak with him about his bill when he comes in for a visit.

c. Send a letter asking him to please call the office. State in the letter that you are worried about him.

d. Flag his record to warn anyone making an appointment for him that he is not to be seen until he pays on his bill.

e. Terminate the physician-patient contract in writing.

49. A coworker tells you that the patient is very rich. She says that he is just getting old and can't keep up with his bills any longer. Circle all appropriate actions in the list below.

a. Tell the coworker to mind her own business.

b. Do not consider this gossip in your dealings with the patient.

c. Contact the patient's next of kin and tell them that he needs help.

d. Send the patient a letter telling him you know he has the funds to pay his bill.

e. Do nothing until you reach the patient.

f. Do not mention this new information when you do speak with him.

PSY PROCEDURE 11-1 Evaluate and Manage a Patient's Account

Name: ______________________ Date: __________ Time: __________ Grade: __________

EQUIPMENT: Simulation including scenario; sample patient ledger card with transactions; yellow, blue, and red stickers (yellow for accounts 30 days past due; blue for accounts 60 days past due; red for accounts 90 days past due). See Work Product 1.

STANDARDS: Given the needed equipment and a place to work the student will perform this skill with _____% accuracy in a total of _____ minutes. *(Your instructor will tell you what the percentage and time limits will be before you begin.)*

KEY: 4 = Satisfactory 0 = Unsatisfactory NA = This step is not counted

PROCEDURE STEPS	SELF	PARTNER	INSTRUCTOR
1. Review the patient's account history to determine the "age" of the account. If payment has not been made between 30 and 59 days from today's date, the account is 40 days past due, and so on.	☐	☐	☐
2. Flag the account for appropriate action. Place a yellow flag (sticker) on accounts that are 30 days old. Place a blue flag on accounts that are 60 days old. Place a red flag on accounts that are 90 days old.	☐	☐	☐
3. Set aside accounts that have had no payment in 91 days or longer.	☐	☐	☐
4. Make copies of the ledger cards.	☐	☐	☐
5. Sort the copies by category: 30, 60, 90 days.	☐	☐	☐
6. Write or stamp the copies with the appropriate message.	☐	☐	☐
7. Mail the statements to the patients.	☐	☐	☐
8. Follow through with the collection process by continually reviewing past due accounts.	☐	☐	☐
9. AFF When you call a patient with a seriously past due account, he informs you that he has not paid because his wife passed away and he cannot hardly get through the day. Explain how you would respond.	☐	☐	☐

____

____

____

____

CALCULATION

Total Possible Points: ______

Total Points Earned: ______ Multiplied by 100 = ______ Divided by Total Possible Points = ______ %

PASS ☐ **FAIL** ☐ **COMMENTS:**

Student's signature ______________________ Date ______

Partner's signature ______________________ Date ______

Instructor's signature ______________________ Date ______

PSY PROCEDURE 11-2 Composing a Collection Letter

Name: ______________________ Date: ________ Time: ________ Grade: ________

EQUIPMENT: Ledger cards generated in Procedure 11-1, word processor, stationery with letterhead

STANDARDS: Given the needed equipment and a place to work the student will perform this skill with _____% accuracy in a total of _____ minutes. *(Your instructor will tell you what the percentage and time limits will be before you begin.)*

KEY: 4 = Satisfactory 0 = Unsatisfactory NA = This step is not counted

PROCEDURE STEPS	SELF	PARTNER	INSTRUCTOR
1. Review the patients' accounts and sort the accounts by age.	☐	☐	☐
2. Design a rough draft of a form letter that can be used for collections.	☐	☐	☐
3. In the first paragraph, tell the patient why you are writing.	☐	☐	☐
4. Inform the patient of the action you expect. For example: "To avoid further action, please pay $50.00 on this account by Friday, May 1, 20__."	☐	☐	☐
5. Proofread the rough draft for errors, clarity, accuracy, and retype.	☐	☐	☐
6. Take the collection letter to a supervisor or physician for approval.	☐	☐	☐
7. Fill in the appropriate amounts and dates on each letter. Ask for at least half of the account balance within a 2-week period.	☐	☐	☐
8. Print, sign, and mail the letter.	☐	☐	☐
9. AFF You are helping a coworker get her collections letters in the mail. You notice several errors in the letters. Explain how you would respond.	☐	☐	☐

CALCULATION

Total Possible Points: ______

Total Points Earned: ______ Multiplied by 100 = ______ Divided by Total Possible Points = ______ %

PASS ☐ **FAIL** ☐ **COMMENTS:**

Student's signature ______________________ Date ______

Partner's signature ______________________ Date ______

Instructor's signature ______________________ Date ______

WORK PRODUCT 1

Grade: ________

PERFORM ACCOUNTS RECEIVABLE PROCEDURES

Your office's billing cycle posts bills on the first of every month. Review the list of outstanding payments and organize in the Aging of Accounts Receivable Report below.

- Oliver Santino visited the office on April 27 for a physical and blood work. The bill was $250.
- Warren Gates visited the office on May 8. His bill was $55.
- Tamara Jones visited the office on June 18 for a physical. The cost for the physical was $125, with an additional $55 for lab work.
- Amir Shell visited the office on June 25 for a physical exam and chest x-rays. The bill was $315.
- Nora Stevenson visited the office on July 9 to have a wound sutured. The bill was $100.

Below is an aging schedule as of August 30, 2012. Fill in the information for these patients. You may enter an account number of 000-00-0000 for all patients.

Aging of Accounts Receivable Report: August 30, 2012

Patient Name	Account Number	Due Date	Amount
Accounts 30 Days Past Due:			
________	________	________	________
________	________	________	________
________	________	________	________
________	________	________	________
________	________	________	________
Accounts 60 Days Past Due:			
________	________	________	________
________	________	________	________
________	________	________	________
________	________	________	________
________	________	________	________
Accounts 90 Days Past Due:			
________	________	________	________
________	________	________	________
________	________	________	________
________	________	________	________
________	________	________	________
Accounts 120 Days or More Past Due:			
________	________	________	________
________	________	________	________
________	________	________	________
________	________	________	________
________	________	________	________
Total Overdue Accounts Receivable			________

WORK PRODUCT 2

Grade: ________

PERFORM BILLING AND COLLECTION PROCEDURES

Caroline Cusick has an outstanding balance of $415 due to the medical office Pediatric Associates, 1415 San Juan Way, Santa Cruz, CA 95060. Write a collection letter to the patient to tell her about her overdue account. Her contact information is as follows: Caroline Cusick, 24 Beach Street, Santa Cruz, CA 95060. Print the letter and attach to this sheet.

CHAPTER

12 Accounting Responsibilities

Learning Outcomes

Cognitive Domain

1. Spell and define the key terms
2. Explain the concept of the pegboard bookkeeping system
3. Describe the components of the pegboard system
4. Identify and discuss the special features of the pegboard daysheet
5. Describe the functions of a computer accounting system
6. List the uses and components of computer accounting reports
7. Explain banking services, including types of accounts and fees
8. Describe the accounting cycle
9. Describe the components of a record-keeping system
10. Explain the process of ordering supplies and paying invoices
11. Explain basic booking computations
12. Differentiate between bookkeeping and accounting
13. Describe banking procedures
14. Discuss predations for accepting checks
15. Compare types of endorsement
16. Differentiate between accounts payable and accounts receivable
17. Compare manual and computerized bookkeeping systems used in ambulatory health care
18. Describe common periodic financial reports
19. Explain billing and payment options
20. Identify procedure for preparing patient accounts
21. Discuss types of adjustments that may be made to a patient's account

Psychomotor Domain

1. Prepare a bank deposit (Procedure 12-9)
2. Perform accounts receivable procedures, including:
   a. Post entries on a daysheet (Procedures 12-1, 12-2)
   b. Perform billing procedures
   c. Perform collection procedures
   d. Post adjustments (Procedure 12-5)
   e. Process a credit balance (Procedure 12-3)
   f. Process refunds (Procedure 12-4)
   g. Post non-sufficient fund (NSF) checks (Procedure 12-7)
   h. Post collection agency payments (Procedure 12-6)
3. Balance a daysheet (Procedure 12-8)
4. Reconcile a bank statement (Procedure 12-10)
5. Maintain a petty cash account (Procedure 12-11)
6. Order supplies (Procedure 12-12)
7. Write a check (Procedure 12-13)

Affective Domain

1. Apply ethical behaviors, including honesty and integrity in performance of medical assisting practice
2. Apply local, state and federal health care legislation and regulation appropriate to the medical assisting practice setting
3. Demonstrate sensitivity and professionalism in handling accounts receivable activities with clients

ABHES Competencies

1. Prepare and reconcile a bank statement and deposit record
2. Post entries on a daysheet
3. Perform billing and collection procedures
4. Perform accounts receivable procedures
5. Use physician fee schedule
6. Establish and maintain a petty cash fund
7. Post adjustments
8. Process credit balance
9. Process refunds
10. Post non-sufficient funds (NSF)
11. Post collection agency payments
12. Use manual or computerized bookkeeping systems

Name: ______________________ Date: __________ Grade: __________

COG MULTIPLE CHOICE

1. The best place to put petty cash is:
   a. in the same drawer as the other cash and checks.
   b. in a separate, secured drawer.
   c. in an envelope stored in the staff room.
   d. in the physician's office.
   e. in a locked supply cabinet.

2. Which of the following information is found on a patient's ledger card?
   a. Date of birth
   b. Social Security number
   c. Blood type
   d. Insurance information
   e. Marital status

3. The purpose of the posting proofs section is to:
   a. enter the day's totals and balance the daysheet.
   b. update and maintain a patient's financial record.
   c. make note of any credit the patient has on file.
   d. make note of any debit the patient has on file.
   e. allow for any adjustments that need to be made.

4. Which of the following might you purchase using petty cash?
   a. Cotton swabs
   b. Thermometer covers
   c. Office supplies
   d. Non-latex gloves
   e. New x-ray machine

Scenario for questions 5 and 6: A new patient comes in and gives you his insurance card. The patient's insurance allows $160.00 for a routine checkup. Of this, insurance will pay 75% of his bill. The actual price of the checkup is $160.00.

5. How much will the patient need to pay?
   a. $0
   b. $40.00
   c. $120.00
   d. $75.00
   e. $160.00

6. How much will the insurance company pay?
   a. $120.00
   b. $40.00
   c. $160.00
   d. $32.00
   e. $0

7. A check register is used to:
   a. hold checks until they are ready for deposit.
   b. create a checklist of daily office duties.
   c. make a list of payments the office is still owed.
   d. record all checks that go in and out of the office.
   e. remind patients when their payments are due.

8. Ideally if you are using a pegboard accounting system, what is the best way to organize your ledgers?
   a. File all ledgers alphabetically in a single tray.
   b. Alphabetically file paid ledgers in one tray and ledgers with outstanding balances in another.
   c. Numerically file paid ledgers in the front of the tray and ledgers with outstanding balances in the back.
   d. Alphabetically file paid ledgers into the patient's folders and ledgers with outstanding balances in a tray.
   e. file all ledgers into the patient's files.

9. Accounts receivable is:
   a. a record of all monies due to the practice.
   b. the people the practice owes money to.
   c. the transactions transferred from a different office.
   d. any outstanding inventory bills.
   e. a list of patients who have paid in the last month.

10. It is unsafe to use credit card account numbers on purchases made:

a. over the phone.

b. by fax.

c. through e-mail.

d. from a catalog.

e. in person.

11. When you have a deposit that includes cash, what is the only way you should get it to the bank?

a. Deliver it by hand.

b. Deliver it into a depository.

c. Send it by mail with enough postage.

d. Deliver checks by mail and cash by hand.

e. Do not accept cash as payment.

12. Which of the following is a benefit of paying bills by computer?

a. You do not need to keep a record of paying your bills.

b. Entering data into the computer is quick and easy.

c. Information can be "memorized" and stored.

d. You can divide columns into groups of expenses (rent, paychecks, etc.).

e. You can easily correct any errors.

13. Most medical offices generally use:

a. standard business checks.

b. certified checks.

c. traveler's checks.

d. money orders.

e. cash deposits.

14. What is a quick way to find order numbers when making a purchase?

a. Check the packing slip of a previous order.

b. Find a previous bill for any item numbers.

c. Check past purchase orders for their order numbers.

d. Call the supplier for a list of item numbers.

e. Look at the supplier's Web site.

15. Summation reports are:

a. lists of all the clients who entered the office.

b. reports that track all expenses and income.

c. computer reports that compile all daily totals.

d. lists that analyze an office's activities.

e. reports the IRS sends an office being audited.

16. Why is the adjustment column so important?

a. It assists you in deciding the discount percentage.

b. It records all transactions a patient has made in your office.

c. It allows you to add discounts and credit to change the total.

d. It keeps track of any changes a patient has in health care.

e. It keeps track of bounced checks.

17. Which of the following is NOT an important reason for performing an office inventory of equipment and supplies?

a. It will help you know when to order new supplies and/or equipment.

b. It will help you calculate how much money you will need to spend on new equipment.

c. It will alert you of any misuse/theft of supplies or equipment.

d. The information will be needed for tax purposes.

e. It will help you see if you will have excess supplies to share with employees.

18. In a bookkeeping system, things of value relating to the practice are called:

a. assets.

b. liabilities.

c. debits.

d. credits.

e. audits.

19. The amount of capital the physician has invested in the practice is referred to as:

a. assets.

b. credits.

c. equity.

d. liabilities.

e. invoices.

20. Overpayments under $5 are generally:

a. sent back to the patient.

b. placed in petty cash.

c. left on the account as a credit.

d. deposited in a special overpayment account.

e. mailed to the insurance company.

COG MATCHING

Grade: _______

Match the following key terms to their definitions.

Key Terms

21. _____ accounting cycle

22. _____ accounts payable

23. _____ adjustment

24. _____ audit

25. _____ balance

26. _____ bookkeeping

27. _____ charge slip

28. _____ check register

29. _____ check stub

30. _____ credit

31. _____ daysheet

32. _____ debit

33. _____ encounter form

34. _____ Internal Revenue Service (IRS)

35. _____ invoice

36. _____ liabilities

37. _____ ledger card

Definitions

a. a preprinted three-part form that can be placed on a daysheet to record the patient's charges and payments along with other information in an encounter form

b. a charge or money owed to an account

c. a record of all money owed to the business

d. a document that accompanies a supply order and lists the enclosed items

e. any report that provides a summary of activities, such as a payroll report or profit-and-loss statement

f. a daily business record of charges and payments

g. a statement of income and expenditures; shows whether in a given period a business made or lost money and how much

h. statement of debt owed; a bill

i. a review of an account

j. a consecutive 12-month period for financial record keeping following either a fiscal year or the calendar year

k. a balance in one's favor on an account; a promise to pay a bill at a later date; record of payment received

l. listing financial transactions in a ledger

m. a continuous record of business transactions with debits and credits

n. change in a posted account

o. a federal agency that regulates and enforces various taxes

p. amount of money a bank or business charges for a check written on an account with insufficient funds

q. amounts of money the practice owes

r. organized and accurate record-keeping system of financial transactions

s. a document that lists required items to be purchased

38. ____ packing slip

39. ____ posting

40. ____ profit-and-loss statement

41. ____ purchase order

42. ____ returned check fee

43. ____ service charge

44. ____ summation report

t. preprinted patient statement that lists codes for basic office charges and has sections to record charges incurred in an office visit, the patient's current balance, and next appointment

u. that which is left over after the additions and subtractions have been made to an account

v. piece of paper that indicates to whom a check was issued, in what amount, and on what date

w. a document used to record the checks that have been written

x. a charge by a bank for various services

COG SHORT ANSWER

Grade: ________

45. What are banking services?

____

____

____

____

46. Why is correction fluid not used in a medical office, and what is the proper procedure to correct a mistake?

____

____

____

____

47. What are four steps you can take if an item you ordered was not delivered?

____

____

____

____

48. List four items that should be readily available in case your office is audited.

49. What is a returned check fee?

50. Why might you run a trial daily report before you run a final daily report?

51. The office you are working in has recently updated its bookkeeping system from pegboard to computer. Now, the physician wants to utilize all the capabilities the new system offers. One particular function that interests her is the computer accounting reports. List the different types of reports and briefly describe their uses.

COG PSY ACTIVE LEARNING

Grade: ___________

52. During a staff meeting, the issue of ordering supplies comes up. The office has been buying small quantities of all supplies, causing some items to quickly run out, while others are stockpiled in disuse. The head physician wants to figure out a way to spend the budget more efficiently, and asks you to be in charge of the next order. What steps can you take to determine which items you will order in the office's next purchase? How can you further improve the office's expenditure?

____

____

____

____

53. Your office currently is using a checking account at a local bank. However, the physician you work for is thinking about changing over to a money market account, because he has heard the interest is much better in a money market account. He knows about an offer through another bank that will waive the minimum balance of $500 for 3 months. What important information should you look into before you give him your opinion? Discuss the differences between a checking account and a money market account, and include the advantages and disadvantages to switching accounts.

____

____

____

____

COG IDENTIFICATION

Grade: ___________

54. There are several advantages of a computerized system over a manual system. Read the selection below, and circle the functions that are computerized accounting functions only.

a. Entries are recorded in a patient's file.

b. Quickly create invoices and receipts.

c. Calculation of each transaction is made, as well as a total at the end of the day.

d. Performs bookkeeping, making appointments, and generating office reports.

e. Daily activities are recorded.

f. Bill reminders are placed to keep track of expenses.

55. A medical office is just starting up, and one of the first things the bookkeeper needs to do is find a bank. Fill in the chart below with descriptions of checking, savings, and money market accounts.

Checking Account	Savings Account	Money Market Account

56. The office you are working in has an accounting cycle that begins in June. Describe what the accounting cycle is, and what kind of year your office follows.

____

____

____

____

57. The office manager ordered a new endorsement stamp from the bank. In the meantime, you need to deposit a check for Rinku Banjere, MD, into account number 123-4567-890. Endorse the check below for deposit.

ENDORSE HERE

____

____

____

DO NOT SIGN/WRITE/STAMP BELOW THIS LINE
FOR FINANCIAL INSTITUTION USE ONLY*

PSY WHAT WOULD YOU DO?

Grade: ________

58. A patient's check has been returned for insufficient funds. The patient asks you to send it back through the bank. What would you do?

____

____

____

____

59. Explain the process of ordering supplies and paying invoices.

____

____

____

____

COG TRUE OR FALSE?

Grade: ________

Determine whether the following statements are true or false. If false, explain why.

60. Once you have entered a patient transaction on the daysheet, you give the ledger to the patient as a receipt.

____

61. As long as your bookkeeping records are accurate and the figures balance, you do not need to save receipts.

____

62. You should always compare the prices and quality of office supplies when you are placing an order.

____

63. Audits are performed in the office yearly by the IRS.

____

64. Packing slips are used by the manufacturer and can be destroyed upon opening a package of supplies.

____

COG PATIENT EDUCATION

Grade: ______

65. Your patient is a young woman who does not understand what happens to the difference between what a physician charges and what her insurance company will pay. In her case, the physician's charge is $100, but insurance only allows for $80. The insurance company will pay for 75% of the cost. How much will the patient pay? Explain to her how this works, and how the charge is determined.

______

______

______

______

AFF CASE STUDY FOR CRITICAL THINKING

Grade: ______

You have been working at a small, one-physician practice for about 2 weeks. You share the front office with the office manager, who has been working there for 20 years. She goes on vacation and in the course of covering some of her duties, you discover suspicious entries in the accounts payable records. You wonder if she is paying her own bills out of the office account.

66. What should you do? Choose all appropriate actions from the list below.

a. Nothing, she is your boss and you are new here.

b. Ask your coworkers for advice.

c. Question her about what you found when she returns.

d. Tell the physician immediately.

e. Tell the physician's wife of your suspicions.

f. Keep it to yourself; it is none of your business.

g. Post the situation on Facebook and ask for advice.

h. Investigate further while she is away by going over all of the check entries.

PSY PROCEDURE 12-1 Post Charges on a Daysheet

Name: ______________________ Date: ________ Time: ________ Grade: ________

EQUIPMENT/SUPPLIES: Pen, pegboard, calculator, daysheet, encounter forms, ledger cards, previous day's balance, list of patients and charges, fee schedule

STANDARDS: Given the needed equipment and a place to work the student will perform this skill with ________% accuracy in a total of ________ minutes. *(Your instructor will tell you what the percentage and time limits will be before you begin.)*

KEY: 4 = Satisfactory 0 = Unsatisfactory NA = This step is not counted

PROCEDURE STEPS	SELF	PARTNER	INSTRUCTOR
1. Place a new daysheet on the pegboard and record the totals from the previous daysheet.	☐	☐	☐
2. Align the patient's ledger card with the first available line on the daysheet.	☐	☐	☐
3. Place the receipt to align with the appropriate line on the ledger card.	☐	☐	☐
4. Record the number of the receipt in the appropriate column.	☐	☐	☐
5. Write the patient's name on the receipt.	☐	☐	☐
6. Record any existing balance the patient owes in the previous balance column of the daysheet.	☐	☐	☐
7. Record a brief description of the charge in the description line.	☐	☐	☐
8. Record the total charges in the charge column. Press hard so that the marks go through to the ledger card and the daysheet.	☐	☐	☐
9. Add the total charges to the previous balance and record in the current balance column.	☐	☐	☐
10. Return the ledger card to appropriate storage.	☐	☐	☐

CALCULATION

Total Possible Points: ______

Total Points Earned: ______ Multiplied by 100 = ______ Divided by Total Possible Points = ______ %

PASS ☐ **FAIL** ☐ **COMMENTS:**

Student's signature ______________________ Date ______

Partner's signature ______________________ Date ______

Instructor's signature ______________________ Date ______

PSY PROCEDURE 12-2 Post Payments on a Daysheet

Name: ______________________ Date: ________ Time: ________ Grade: ________

EQUIPMENT/SUPPLIES: Pen, pegboard, calculator, daysheet, encounter forms, ledger cards, previous day's balance, list of patients and charges, fee schedule

COMPUTER AND MEDICAL OFFICE SOFTWARE: Follow the software requirements for posting credits to patient accounts.

STANDARDS: Given the needed equipment and a place to work the student will perform this skill with ______% accuracy in a total of ______ minutes. *(Your instructor will tell you what the percentage and time limits will be before you begin.)*

KEY: 4 = Satisfactory 0 = Unsatisfactory NA =This step is not counted

PROCEDURE STEPS	SELF	PARTNER	INSTRUCTOR
1. Place a new daysheet on the pegboard and record the totals from the previous daysheet.	☐	☐	☐
2. Align the patient's ledger card with the first available line on the daysheet.	☐	☐	☐
3. Place receipt to align with the appropriate line on the ledger card.	☐	☐	☐
4. Record the number of the receipt in the appropriate column.	☐	☐	☐
5. Write the patient's name on the receipt.	☐	☐	☐
6. Record any existing balance the patient owes in the previous balance column of the daysheet.	☐	☐	☐
7. Record the source and type of the payment in the description line.	☐	☐	☐
8. Record appropriate adjustments in adjustment column.	☐	☐	☐
9. Record the total payment in the payment column. Press hard so that marks go through to the ledger card and the daysheet.	☐	☐	☐
10. Subtract the payment and adjustments from the outstanding/ previous balance, and record the current balance.	☐	☐	☐
11. Return the ledger card to appropriate storage.	☐	☐	☐

CALCULATION

Total Possible Points: ______

Total Points Earned: ______ Multiplied by 100 = ______ Divided by Total Possible Points = ______ %

PASS ☐ **FAIL** ☐ **COMMENTS:**

Student's signature ______________________ Date ______

Partner's signature ______________________ Date ______

Instructor's signature ______________________ Date ______

PSY PROCEDURE 12-3 Process a Credit Balance

Name: ______________ Date: ________ Time: ________ Grade: ________

EQUIPMENT/SUPPLIES: Pen, pegboard, calculator, daysheet, ledger card

STANDARDS: Given the needed equipment and a place to work the student will perform this skill with ______% accuracy in a total of ______ minutes. *(Your instructor will tell you what the percentage and time limits will be before you begin.)*

KEY: 4 = Satisfactory 0 = Unsatisfactory NA =This step is not counted

PROCEDURE STEPS	SELF	PARTNER	INSTRUCTOR
1. Determine the reason for the credit balance.	☐	☐	☐
2. Place brackets around the balance indicating that it is a negative number.	☐	☐	☐
3. Write a refund check and follow the steps in Procedure 12-7.	☐	☐	☐

CALCULATION

Total Possible Points: ______

Total Points Earned: ______ Multiplied by 100 = ______ Divided by Total Possible Points = ______ %

PASS ☐ **FAIL** ☐ **COMMENTS:**

Student's signature ______________ Date ______

Partner's signature ______________ Date ______

Instructor's signature ______________ Date ______

PSY PROCEDURE 12-4 Process Refunds

Name: ______________________ Date: ________ Time: ________ Grade: ________

EQUIPMENT/SUPPLIES: Pen, pegboard, calculator, daysheet, ledger card, checkbook, check register, word processor letterhead, envelope, postage, copy machine, patient's chart, refund file

STANDARDS: Given the needed equipment and a place to work the student will perform this skill with ______% accuracy in a total of ______ minutes. *(Your instructor will tell you what the percentage and time limits will be before you begin.)*

KEY: 4 = Satisfactory 0 = Unsatisfactory NA =This step is not counted

PROCEDURE STEPS	SELF	PARTNER	INSTRUCTOR
1. Determine who gets the refund, the patient or the insurance company.	☐	☐	☐
2. Pull patient's ledger card and place on current daysheet aligned with the first available line.	☐	☐	☐
3. Post the amount of the refund in the adjustment column in brackets indicating it is a debit, not a credit, adjustment.	☐	☐	☐
4. Write "Refund to Patient" or "Refund to _____" (name of insurance company) in the description column.	☐	☐	☐
5. Write a check for the credit amount made out to the appropriate party.	☐	☐	☐
6. Record the amount and name of payee in the check register.	☐	☐	☐
7. Mail check with letter of explanation to patient or insurance company.	☐	☐	☐
8. Place copy of check and copy of letter in the patient's record or in refund file.	☐	☐	☐
9. Return the patient's ledger card to its storage area.	☐	☐	☐

CALCULATION

Total Possible Points: ______

Total Points Earned: ______ Multiplied by 100 = ______ Divided by Total Possible Points = ______ %

PASS ☐ **FAIL** ☐ **COMMENTS:**

Student's signature ______________________ Date ______

Partner's signature ______________________ Date ______

Instructor's signature ______________________ Date ______

PSY PROCEDURE 12-5 Post Adjustments to a Daysheet

Name: ______________________ Date: ________ Time: ________ Grade: ________

EQUIPMENT/SUPPLIES: Pen, pegboard, calculator, daysheet, encounter forms, ledger cards, previous day's balance, list of patients and charges, fee schedule

COMPUTER AND MEDICAL OFFICE SOFTWARE: Follow the software requirements for posting credits to patient accounts.

STANDARDS: Given the needed equipment and a place to work the student will perform this skill with ______% accuracy in a total of ______ minutes. *(Your instructor will tell you what the percentage and time limits will be before you begin.)*

KEY: 4 = Satisfactory 0 = Unsatisfactory NA =This step is not counted

PROCEDURE STEPS	SELF	PARTNER	INSTRUCTOR
1. Pull patient's ledger card and place on current daysheet aligned with the first available line.	☐	☐	☐
2. Post the amount to be written off in the adjustment column in brackets indicating it is a debit, not a credit, adjustment.	☐	☐	☐
3. Subtract the adjustment from the outstanding/previous balance, and record in the current balance column.	☐	☐	☐
4. Return the ledger card to appropriate storage.	☐	☐	☐

CALCULATION

Total Possible Points: ______

Total Points Earned: ______ Multiplied by 100 = ______ Divided by Total Possible Points = ______ %

PASS ☐ **FAIL** ☐ **COMMENTS:**

Student's signature ______________________ Date ______

Partner's signature ______________________ Date ______

Instructor's signature ______________________ Date ______

PSY PROCEDURE 12-6 Post Collection Agency Payments

Name: ______________________ Date: __________ Time: __________ Grade: __________

EQUIPMENT/SUPPLIES: Pen, pegboard, calculator, daysheet, patient's ledger card

STANDARDS: Given the needed equipment and a place to work the student will perform this skill with ______% accuracy in a total of ______ minutes. *(Your instructor will tell you what the percentage and time limits will be before you begin.)*

KEY: 4 = Satisfactory 0 = Unsatisfactory NA =This step is not counted

PROCEDURE STEPS	SELF	PARTNER	INSTRUCTOR
1. Review check stub or report from the collection agency explaining the amounts to be applied to the accounts.	☐	☐	☐
2. Pull the patients' ledger cards.	☐	☐	☐
3. Post the amount to be applied in the payment column for each patient.	☐	☐	☐
4. Adjust off the amount representing the percentage of the payment charged by the collection agency.	☐	☐	☐

CALCULATION

Total Possible Points: ______

Total Points Earned: ______ Multiplied by 100 = ______ Divided by Total Possible Points = ______ %

PASS ☐ **FAIL** ☐ **COMMENTS:**

Student's signature ______________________ Date ______

Partner's signature ______________________ Date ______

Instructor's signature ______________________ Date ______

PSY PROCEDURE 12-7 Process NSF Checks

Name: ______________________ Date: ________ Time: ________ Grade: ________

EQUIPMENT/SUPPLIES: Pen, pegboard, calculator, daysheet, patient's ledger card

STANDARDS: Given the needed equipment and a place to work the student will perform this skill with ______% accuracy in a total of ______ minutes. *(Your instructor will tell you what the percentage and time limits will be before you begin.)*

KEY: 4 = Satisfactory 0 = Unsatisfactory NA = This step is not counted

PROCEDURE STEPS	SELF	PARTNER	INSTRUCTOR
1. Pull patient's ledger card and place on current daysheet aligned with the first available line.	☐	☐	☐
2. Write the amount of the check in the payment column in brackets indicating it is a debit, not a credit, adjustment.	☐	☐	☐
3. Write "Check Returned For Nonsufficient Funds" in the description column.	☐	☐	☐
4. Post a returned check charge with an appropriate explanation in the charge column.	☐	☐	☐
5. Write "Bank Fee for Returned Check" in the description column.	☐	☐	☐
6. Call the patient to advise him of the returned check and the fee.	☐	☐	☐
7. Construct a proper letter of explanation and a copy of the ledger card and mail to patient.	☐	☐	☐
8. Place a copy of the letter and the check in the patient's file.	☐	☐	☐
9. Make arrangements for the patient to pay cash.	☐	☐	☐
10. Flag the patient's account as a credit risk for future transactions.	☐	☐	☐
11. Return the patient's ledger card to its storage area.	☐	☐	☐
12. AFF You see a patient whose check was returned for nonsufficient funds out at a soccer game. He whispers to you to keep quiet about the bad check. Explain how you would respond.	☐	☐	☐

____

____

____

____

CALCULATION

Total Possible Points: ______

Total Points Earned: ______ Multiplied by 100 = ______ Divided by Total Possible Points = ______ %

PASS ☐ **FAIL** ☐ **COMMENTS:**

Student's signature ______________________________ Date ______

Partner's signature ______________________________ Date ______

Instructor's signature ______________________________ Date ______

PSY PROCEDURE 12-8 Balance a Daysheet

Name: ______________________ Date: ________ Time: ________ Grade: ________

EQUIPMENT/SUPPLIES: Daysheet with totals brought forward, simulated exercise, calculator, pen

STANDARDS: Given the needed equipment and a place to work the student will perform this skill with ______% accuracy in a total of ______ minutes. *(Your instructor will tell you what the percentage and time limits will be before you begin.)*

KEY: 4 = Satisfactory 0 = Unsatisfactory NA =This step is not counted

PROCEDURE STEPS	SELF	PARTNER	INSTRUCTOR
1. Be sure the totals from the previous daysheet are recorded in the column for previous totals.	☐	☐	☐
2. Total the charge column and place that number in the proper blank.	☐	☐	☐
3. Total the payment column and place that number in the proper blank.	☐	☐	☐
4. Total the adjustment column and place that number in the proper blank.	☐	☐	☐
5. Total the current balance column and place that number in the proper blank.	☐	☐	☐
6. Total the previous balance column and place that number in the proper blank.	☐	☐	☐
7. Add today's totals to the previous totals.	☐	☐	☐
8. Take the grand total of the previous balances, add the grand total of the charges, and subtract the grand total of the payments and adjustments. This number must equal the grand total of the current balance.	☐	☐	☐
9. If the numbers do not match, calculate your totals again, and continue looking for errors until the numbers match. This will prove that the daysheet is balanced, and there are no errors.	☐	☐	☐
10. Record the totals of the columns in the proper space on the next daysheet. You will be prepared for balancing the new daysheet.	☐	☐	☐

CALCULATION

Total Possible Points: ______

Total Points Earned: ______ Multiplied by 100 = ______ Divided by Total Possible Points = ______ %

PASS ☐ **FAIL** ☐ **COMMENTS:**

Student's signature ______________________ Date ______

Partner's signature ______________________ Date ______

Instructor's signature ______________________ Date ______

PSY PROCEDURE 12-9 Complete a Bank Deposit Slip and Make a Deposit

Name: ______________________ Date: __________ Time: __________ Grade: __________

EQUIPMENT/SUPPLIES: Calculator with tape, currency, coins, checks for deposit, deposit slip, endorsement stamp, deposit envelope

STANDARDS: Given the needed equipment and a place to work the student will perform this skill with _______% accuracy in a total of _______ minutes. *(Your instructor will tell you what the percentage and time limits will be before you begin.)*

KEY: 4 = Satisfactory 0 = Unsatisfactory NA = This step is not counted

PROCEDURE STEPS	SELF	PARTNER	INSTRUCTOR
1. Arrange bills face up and sort with the largest denomination on top.	☐	☐	☐
2. Record the total in the cash block on the deposit slip	☐	☐	☐
3. Endorse the back of each check with "For Deposit Only."	☐	☐	☐
4. Record the amount of each check beside an identifying number on the deposit slip.	☐	☐	☐
5. Total and record the amounts of checks in the total of checks line on the deposit slip.	☐	☐	☐
6. Total and record the amount of cash and the amount of checks.	☐	☐	☐
7. Record the total amount of the deposit in the office checkbook register.	☐	☐	☐
8. Make a copy of both sides of the deposit slip for office records.	☐	☐	☐
9. Place the cash, checks, and the completed deposit slip in an envelope or bank bag for transporting to the bank for deposit.	☐	☐	☐

CALCULATION

Total Possible Points: _______

Total Points Earned: _______ Multiplied by 100 = _______ Divided by Total Possible Points = _______ %

PASS ☐ **FAIL** ☐ **COMMENTS:**

Student's signature ______________________________ Date _______

Partner's signature ______________________________ Date _______

Instructor's signature ______________________________ Date _______

PSY PROCEDURE 12-10 Reconcile a Bank Statement

Name: ______________________ Date: ________ Time: ________ Grade: ________

EQUIPMENT/SUPPLIES: Simulated bank statement, reconciliation worksheet, calculator, pen

STANDARDS: Given the needed equipment and a place to work the student will perform this skill with ______% accuracy in a total of ______ minutes. *(Your instructor will tell you what the percentage and time limits will be before you begin.)*

KEY: 4 = Satisfactory 0 = Unsatisfactory NA =This step is not counted

PROCEDURE STEPS	SELF	PARTNER	INSTRUCTOR
1. Compare the opening balance on the new statement with the closing balance on the previous statement.	☐	☐	☐
2. List the bank balance in the appropriate space on the reconciliation worksheet.	☐	☐	☐
3. Compare the check entries on the statement with the entries in the check register.	☐	☐	☐
4. Determine if there are any outstanding checks.	☐	☐	☐
5. Total outstanding checks.	☐	☐	☐
6. Subtract from the checkbook balance items such as withdrawals, automatic payments, or service charges that appeared on the statement but not in the checkbook.	☐	☐	☐
7. Add to the bank statement balance any deposits not shown on the bank statement.	☐	☐	☐
8. Make sure balance in the checkbook and the bank statement agree.	☐	☐	☐

CALCULATION

Total Possible Points: ______

Total Points Earned: ______ Multiplied by 100 = ______ Divided by Total Possible Points = ______ %

PASS ☐ **FAIL** ☐ **COMMENTS:**

Student's signature ______________________ Date ______

Partner's signature ______________________ Date ______

Instructor's signature ______________________ Date ______

PSY PROCEDURE 12-11 Maintain a Petty Cash Account

Name: ______________________ Date: __________ Time: __________ Grade: __________

EQUIPMENT/SUPPLIES: Cash box, play money, checkbook, simulated receipts, and/or vouchers representing expenditures

STANDARDS: Given the needed equipment and a place to work the student will perform this skill with _____% accuracy in a total of _____ minutes. *(Your instructor will tell you what the percentage and time limits will be before you begin.)*

KEY: 4 = Satisfactory 0 = Unsatisfactory NA =This step is not counted

PROCEDURE STEPS	SELF	PARTNER	INSTRUCTOR
1. Count the money remaining in the box.	☐	☐	☐
2. Total the amounts of all vouchers in the petty cash box and determine the amount of expenditures.	☐	☐	☐
3. Subtract the amount of receipts from the original amount in petty cash, to equal the amount of cash remaining in the box.	☐	☐	☐
4. Balance the cash against the receipts.	☐	☐	☐
5. Write a check only for the amount that was used.	☐	☐	☐
6. Record totals on the memo line of the check stub.	☐	☐	☐
7. Sort and record all vouchers to the appropriate accounts.	☐	☐	☐
8. File the list of vouchers and attached receipts.	☐	☐	☐
9. Place cash in petty cash fund.	☐	☐	☐
10. AFF A co-worker asks to borrow money from petty cash for bus fair home. She promises to pay it back tomorrow. Explain how you would respond.	☐	☐	☐

____

____

____

____

CALCULATION

Total Possible Points: _______

Total Points Earned: _______ Multiplied by 100 = _______ Divided by Total Possible Points = _______ %

PASS ☐ **FAIL** ☐ **COMMENTS:**

Student's signature ______________________ Date _______

Partner's signature ______________________ Date _______

Instructor's signature ______________________ Date _______

PSY PROCEDURE 12-12 Order Supplies

Name: ______________________ Date: ________ Time: ________ Grade: ________

EQUIPMENT/SUPPLIES: 5 × 7 index cards, file box with divider cards, computer with Internet (optional), medical supply catalogues

STANDARDS: Given the needed equipment and a place to work the student will perform this skill with _____% accuracy in a total of _____ minutes. *(Your instructor will tell you what the percentage and time limits will be before you begin.)*

KEY: 4 = Satisfactory 0 = Unsatisfactory NA =This step is not counted

PROCEDURE STEPS	SELF	PARTNER	INSTRUCTOR
1. Create a list of supplies to be ordered that is based on inventory done by employees.	☐	☐	☐
2. Create an index card for each supply on the list including the name of the supply in the top left corner, the name and contact information of vendor(s), and product identification number.	☐	☐	☐
3. File the index cards in the file box with divider cards alphabetically or by product type.	☐	☐	☐
4. Record the current price of the item and how the item is supplied.	☐	☐	☐
5. Record the reorder point.	☐	☐	☐

CALCULATION

Total Possible Points: _____

Total Points Earned: _____ Multiplied by 100 = _____ Divided by Total Possible Points = _____ %

PASS ☐ **FAIL** ☐ **COMMENTS:**

Student's signature ______________________ Date _____

Partner's signature ______________________ Date _____

Instructor's signature ______________________ Date _____

PSY PROCEDURE 12-13 Write a Check

Name: ______________________ Date: ________ Time: ________ Grade: ________

EQUIPMENT/SUPPLIES: Simulated page of checks from checkbook, scenario giving amount of check, check register

STANDARDS: Given the needed equipment and a place to work the student will perform this skill with ______% accuracy in a total of ______ minutes. *(Your instructor will tell you what the percentage and time limits will be before you begin.)*

KEY: 4 = Satisfactory 0 = Unsatisfactory NA =This step is not counted

PROCEDURE STEPS	SELF	PARTNER	INSTRUCTOR
1. Fill out the check register with the following information: **a.** check number **b.** date **c.** payee information **d.** amount **e.** previous balance **f.** new balance	☐	☐	☐
2. Enter date on check.	☐	☐	☐
3. Enter payee on check.	☐	☐	☐
4. Enter the amount of check using numerals.	☐	☐	☐
5. Write out the amount of the check beginning as far left as possible and make a straight line to fill in space between dollars and cents.	☐	☐	☐
6. Record cents as a fraction with 100 as the denominator.	☐	☐	☐
7. Obtain appropriate signature(s).	☐	☐	☐
8. Proofread for accuracy.	☐	☐	☐

CALCULATION

Total Possible Points: ______

Total Points Earned: ______ Multiplied by 100 = ______ Divided by Total Possible Points = ______ %

PASS ☐ **FAIL** ☐ **COMMENTS:**

Student's signature ______________________ Date ______

Partner's signature ______________________ Date ______

Instructor's signature ______________________ Date ______

WORK PRODUCT 1

Grade: ________

Perform an Inventory of Supplies

When you are working in a medical office, you may need to keep an inventory of all supplies. The inventory will help you decide when to order new supplies. It will also help you calculate how much money you will need to spend on supplies. Supplies are those items that are consumed quickly and need to be reordered on a regular basis.

If you are currently working in a medical office, use the form below to take an inventory of the supplies in the office. If you do not have access to a medical office, complete an inventory of the supplies in your kitchen or bathroom at home.

Third Street
Physician's Office, Inc.
123 Main Street
Baltimore, MD 21201
410-895-6214

Supply Inventory

Item Description	Item Number or Code	Number Needed in Stock	Number Currently in Stock	Date Ordered	Number Ordered	Unit Price	Total	Actual Delivery Date

WORK PRODUCT 2

Grade: ________

Perform an Inventory of Equipment

When you are working in a medical office, you may need to keep an inventory of all equipment. The inventory will help you decide when to order new equipment. It will also help you calculate how much money you will need to spend on new equipment. Equipment includes items that can be used over and over and generally last many years.

If you are currently working in a medical office, use the form below to take an inventory of the equipment in the office. If you do not have access to a medical office, complete an inventory of the equipment in your kitchen or bathroom at home.

Third Street
Physician's Office, Inc.
123 Main Street
Baltimore, MD 21201
410-895-6214

Equipment Inventory

Item Description	Item Number or Code	Purchase Date	Condition	Comments	Expected New Purchase Date	Cost if Purchased This Year

WORK PRODUCT 3

Grade: ________

Process a Credit Balance

Mr. Juan Rodriguez has switched to a different insurance company. His co-pay with his old carrier was $35 per visit. His new co-pay is $20 per visit. However, there was a billing oversight and Mr. Rodriguez paid his old co-pay. Process Mr. Rodriguez's credit balance on the daysheet.

			CREDITS				
Date	Description	Charges	Payments	Adjust ments	Current Balance	Previous Balance	NAME

Totals This Page					
Totals Previous Page					
Month-To-Date Totals					

WORK PRODUCT 4

Grade: ________

Process a Refund

Mr. Rodriguez has a credit balance of $15 on his account. You need to mail him a refund check. Post this transaction on the daysheet.

			CREDITS				
Date	Description	Charges	Payments	Adjust ments	Current Balance	Previous Balance	NAME

Totals This Page					
Totals Previous Page					
Month-To-Date Totals					

WORK PRODUCT 5

Grade: ________

Post Adjustments

Mr. Rodriguez visits your office for an x-ray of his knee. Your office normally charges $225 for a knee x-ray. However, your physician is a participating provider for Mr. Rodriguez's insurance carrier. His insurance pays your office only $175 for a knee x-ray. Post the proper adjustment on the daysheet.

			CREDITS				
Date	Description	Charges	Payments	Adjust ments	Current Balance	Previous Balance	NAME

Totals This Page					
Totals Previous Page					
Month-To-Date Totals					

WORK PRODUCT 6

Grade: ______

Post NSF Checks

You have just received a check that was returned for nonsufficient funds. The check was written by Martha Montgomery for $750. Post the proper information on the daysheet.

			CREDITS				
Date	Description	Charges	Payments	Adjust ments	Current Balance	Previous Balance	NAME

Totals This Page					
Totals Previous Page					
Month-To-Date Totals					

WORK PRODUCT 7

Grade: ________

Post Collection Agency Payments

You receive a check for $787.50 and the following statement from your collection agency.
Jones & Jones Collections
Account:d. Larsen, MD

Debtor	Amount Collected	Fee	Balance
Martha Montgomery	$750.00	$187.50	$562.50
Johan Johansen	$300.00	$75.00	$225.00
		Total	$787.50

Post the payments to the daysheet.

			CREDITS				
Date	Description	Charges	Payments	Adjust ments	Current Balance	Previous Balance	NAME

Totals This Page					
Totals Previous Page					
Month-To-Date Totals					

WORK PRODUCT 8

Grade: ________

Posting Payments from Medicare

On a blank daysheet provided, post the following Medicare payments. You will need to calculate the adjustments by subtracting the amount allowed from the amount charged. The patient's previous balance will be the amount charged back on the date of service.

Keep in mind that on an actual MEOB, the CPT-4 codes would be used instead of OV, x-ray, etc.

MEDICARE EXPLANATION OF BENEFITS

Name	Charges	Date of Service	Amount Allowed	Amount Paid to Provider	Patient's Responsibility
Smith, John	OV 40.00	3-2-xx	18.00	14.40	3.60
Jones, Anne	OV 100.00 Lab 50.00	3-2-xx	65.00 50.00	52.00 40.00	13.00 10.00
Total:	150.00		115.00	92.00	23.00
Stevens, Sally	OV 150.00 X-ray 200.00	3-2-xx	120.00 160.00	96.00 128.00	24.00 32.00
Total:	350.00		280.00	224.00	56.00
Reynolds, Susan	Consult 300.00	3-2-xx	250.00	200.00	50.00

CREDITS

Date	Description	Charges	Payments	Adjust ments	Current Balance	Previous Balance	NAME

Totals This Page					
Totals Previous Page					
Month-To-Date Totals					

WORK PRODUCT 9

Grade: ________

Putting It All Together

On a blank daysheet provided, complete 1–8.
Post the following transactions on the daysheet provided. Use today's date.

1. Stanley Gleber came in and paid $25.00 in cash on his account. His previous balance is $100.00.

2. Lisa Moore sent a check in the mail for $100.00 to be paid on her account, which carries a balance of $500.00.

3. Elaine Newman came in and handed you a check she received from Blue Cross Blue Shield for $700.00 to be paid on her account, which has a balance of $900.00. The explanation attached to the check indicates it is for surgery she had on 3-1-09. Your physician does NOT participate with Blue Cross Blue Shield. Post the payment with an appropriate description. Will there be an adjustment?

4. Madeline Bell saw the doctor and brings out an encounter form with a charge for an office visit at $50.00 and lab at $150.00. Post her charges. She does not pay today. Her previous balance was zero.

5. Post the collection agency payment for John Simms. His account with a balance of $250.00 was turned over to Equifax on 03/01/12. They collected the entire amount. You receive a check from Equifax. They charge 30% of what they collect, so the check is for 200.00. His balance was not written off when turned over to Equifax, so his previous balance should be 250.00.

6. Hazel Wilbourne paid her charges of $200.00 in full at her last visit. Now you receive a check from Aetna for that visit. The check is for $130.00. Your physician participates with this insurance company, which means he agrees to accept what they pay. In other words, you will not bill the patient for the difference. Post the check to Ms. Wilbourne's account.

7. Ms. Wilbourne now has a credit balance. You will need to send her a check from the office account as a refund. Post the appropriate entry for this transaction. In accounting, a credit balance is put in angle brackets: <200.00>.

8. Calculate and record each column total. Make sure the columns balance by starting with your previous balance, adding the charges, subtracting the payments and adjustments, and this should give you the total of your current balance column. Remember, brackets in accounting mean that you do the opposite when adding your columns, so instead of adding a credit balance when totaling, you will subtract it.

		CREDITS					
Date	Description	Charges	Payments	Adjust ments	Current Balance	Previous Balance	NAME

Totals This Page					
Totals Previous Page					
Month-To-Date Totals					

WORK PRODUCT 10

Grade: __________

Prepare a Bank Deposit

Prepare a bank deposit for the following:

- check for $750 from Martin Montgomery
- check for $35 from Rita Gonzalez
- $125 cash

Use fictitious demographic information for the account holder on the deposit slip.

Newtown Bank, N.A.

DEPOSIT

Name and account number will be verifi ed when presented.

Name	Date
Address	
Signature	Sign here only if cash is received from deposit

ITEMS DEPOSITED	DOLLARS	CENTS
Currency		.
Coin		.
Checks 1		.
2		.
3		.
4		.
Sub Total		.
Less Cash		.
Total Deposit		

Store Number (Commercial Accounts Only) *

Account Number (For CAP Accounts, use 10-digit number.) *

$.

CHAPTER 13

Health Insurance and Reimbursement

Learning Outcomes

Cognitive Domain

1. Spell and define the key terms
2. Identify types of insurance plans
3. Discuss workers' compensation as it applies to patients
4. Identify models of managed care
5. Describe procedures for implementing both managed care and insurance plans
6. Discuss utilization review principles
7. Discuss referral process for patients in a managed care program
8. Describe how guidelines are used in processing an insurance claim
9. Compare processes for filing insurance claims both manually and electronically
10. Describe guidelines for third-party claims
11. Discuss types of physician fee schedules
12. Describe the concept of resource-based relative value scale (RBRVS)
13. Define diagnosis-related groups (DRGs)
14. Name two legal issues affecting claims submissions

Psychomotor Domain

1. Complete a CMS-1500 claim form (Procedure 13-1)
2. Apply both managed care policies and procedures
3. Apply third-party guidelines
4. Complete insurance claim forms
5. Obtain precertification, including documentation
6. Verify eligibility for managed care services

Affective Domain

1. Demonstrate assertive communication with managed care and/or insurance providers
2. Demonstrate sensitivity in communicating with both providers and patients
3. Communicate in language the patient can understand regarding managed care and insurance plans
4. Apply ethical behaviors, including honesty/integrity in performance of medical assisting practice

ABHES Competencies

1. Prepare and submit insurance claims
2. Serve as liaison between physician and others
3. Comply with federal, state and local health laws and regulations

Name: ____________________ Date: ____________ Grade: ____________

COG MULTIPLE CHOICE

1. Which of the following is frequently not covered in group health benefits packages?
   a. Birth control
   b. Childhood immunizations
   c. Routine diagnostic care
   d. Treatment for substance abuse
   e. Regular physical examinations

2. Any payment for medical services that is not paid by the patient or physician is said to be paid by a(n):
   a. second-party payer.
   b. first-party payer.
   c. insurance party payer.
   d. third-party payer.
   e. health care party payer.

3. The criteria a patient must meet for a group benefit plan to provide coverage are called:
   a. eligibility requirements.
   b. patient requirements.
   c. benefit plan requirements.
   d. physical requirements.
   e. insurance requirements.

4. Eligibility for a dependent requires that he or she is:
   a. unmarried.
   b. employed.
   c. living with the employee.
   d. younger than 18.
   e. an excellent student.

5. Whom should you contact about the eligibility of a patient for the health benefits plan?
   a. Claims administrator
   b. Claims investigator
   c. Insurance salesperson
   d. Insurance reviewer
   e. Claims insurer

Scenario for questions 6 and 7: Aziz pays premiums directly to the insurance company, and the insurance company reimburses him for eligible medical expenses.

6. What type of insurance does Aziz have?
   a. Individual health benefits
   b. Public health benefits
   c. Managed care
   d. PPO
   e. HMO

7. Which of the following is likely true of Aziz's insurance?
   a. The insurance is provided by his employer.
   b. Money can be put aside into accounts used for medical expenses.
   c. There are certain restrictions for some illnesses and injuries.
   d. All providers are under contract with the insurer.
   e. There are two levels of benefits in the health plan.

8. An optional health benefits program offered to persons signing up for Social Security benefits is:
   a. Medicare Part A.
   b. Medicare Part B.
   c. Medicaid.
   d. TRICARE/CHAMPVA.
   e. HMO.

9. After the deductible has been met, what percentage of the approved charges does Medicare reimburse to the physician?
   a. 0
   b. 20
   c. 75
   d. 80
   e. 100

10. Which benefits program bases eligibility on a patient's eligibility for other state programs such as welfare assistance?

- **a.** Workers' Compensation
- **b.** Medicare
- **c.** Medicaid
- **d.** TRICARE/CHAMPVA
- **e.** Social Security

11. Which of the following is a medical expense that Medicaid provides 100% coverage for?

- **a.** Family planning
- **b.** Colorectal screening
- **c.** Bone density testing
- **d.** Pap smears
- **e.** Mammograms

12. In a traditional insurance plan:

- **a.** the covered patient may seek care from any provider.
- **b.** the insurer has no relationship with the provider.
- **c.** a patient can be admitted to a hospital only if that admission has been certified by the insurer.
- **d.** there is no third-party payer.
- **e.** the patient cannot be billed for the deductible.

13. Which of the following is a plan typically developed by hospitals and physicians to attract patients?

- **a.** HMO
- **b.** PPO
- **c.** HSA
- **d.** TPA
- **e.** UCR

14. Which of the following is true about both HMOs and PPOs?

- **a.** Both allow patients to see any physician of their choice and receive benefits.
- **b.** Both contract directly with participating providers, hospitals, and physicians.
- **c.** Both offer benefits at two levels, commonly referred to as *in-network* and *out-of-network*.
- **d.** Both are not risk-bearing and do not have any financial involvement in the health plan.
- **e.** Both incorporate independent practice associations.

15. Which of the following is a government-sponsored health benefits plan?

- **a.** TRICARE/CHAMPVA
- **b.** HMO
- **c.** HSA
- **d.** PPO
- **e.** PHO

16. If a provider is unethical, you should:

- **a.** correct the issue yourself.
- **b.** immediately stop working for the provider.
- **c.** comply with all requests to misrepresent medical records but report the physician.
- **d.** do whatever the physician asks to avoid confrontation.
- **e.** explain that you are legally bound to truthful billing, and report the physician.

17. A patient's ID card:

- **a.** contains the information needed to file a claim on it.
- **b.** should be updated at least once every 2 years.
- **c.** must be cleared before an emergency can be treated.
- **d.** is updated and sent to Medicaid patients bimonthly.
- **e.** is not useful for determining if the patient is a dependent.

18. What information is needed to fill out a CMS-1500 claim form?

- **a.** A copy of the patient's chart
- **b.** Location where patient will be recovering
- **c.** Diagnostic codes from encounter form
- **d.** Copies of hospitalization paperwork
- **e.** Physician's record and degree

19. Claims that are submitted electronically:

a. violate HIPAA standards.

b. contain fewer errors than those that are mailed.

c. require approval from the patient.

d. increase costs for Medicare patients.

e. reduce the reimbursement cycle.

20. Normally, coverage has an amount below which services are not reimbursable. This is referred to as the:

a. deductible.

b. coinsurance.

c. balance billing.

d. benefits.

e. claim.

21. Which is true about how a managed care system is different from a traditional insurance coverage system?

a. They usually are less costly.

b. They cost more but have more benefits.

c. They cost the same but have more benefits.

d. You can only use network physicians.

COG MATCHING

Grade: ______

Match the following key terms to their definitions.

Key Terms

22. ____ assignment of benefits

23. ____ balance billing

24. ____ capitation

25. ____ carrier

26. ____ claims administrator

27. ____ co-insurance

28. ____ coordination of benefits

29. ____ co-payments

30. ____ crossover claim

31. ____ deductible

32. ____ dependent

33. ____ eligibility

34. ____ explanation of benefits (EOB)

Definitions

a. an individual who manages the third-party reimbursement policies for a medical practice

b. the part of the payment for a service that a patient must pay

c. the determination of an insured's right to receive benefits from a third-party payer based on criteria such as payment of premiums

d. spouse, children, and sometimes other individuals designated by the insured who are covered under a health care plan

e. the transfer of the patient's legal right to collect third-party benefits to the provider of the services

f. a company that assumes the risk of an insurance company

g. a group of physicians and specialists that conducts a review of a disputed case and makes a final recommendation

h. an organization that provides a wide range of services through a contract with a specified group at a predetermined payment

i. billing the patients for the difference between the physician's charges and the Medicare-approved charges

j. an organization of nongroup physicians developed to allow independent physicians to compete with prepaid group practices

k. a coalition of physicians and a hospital contracting with large employers, insurance carriers, and other benefits groups to provide discounted health services

35. _____ fee-for-service

36. _____ fee schedule

37. _____ group member

38. _____ healthcare savings account (HSA)

39. _____ health maintenance organization (HMO)

40. _____ independent practice association (IPA)

41. _____ managed care

42. _____ Medicare

43. _____ peer review organization

44. _____ physician hospital organization

45. _____ preferred provider organization (PPO)

46. _____ usual, customary, and reasonable (UCR)

47. _____ utilization review

l. an established set of fees charged for specific services and paid by the patient or insurance carrier

m. the practice of third-party payers to control costs by requiring physicians to adhere to specific rules as a condition of payment

n. the method of designating the order in multiple-carriers pay benefits to avoid duplication of payment

o. a statement from an insurance carrier that outlines which services are being paid

p. a government-sponsored health benefits package that provides insurance for the elderly

q. a claim that moves over automatically from one coverage to another for payment

r. a policyholder who is covered by a group insurance carrier

s. a type of health benefit program whose purpose is to contract with providers, then lease this network of contracted providers to health care plans

t. an employee benefit that allows individuals to save money through payroll deduction to accounts that can be used only for medical care

u. a list of pre-established fee allowances set for specific services performed by a provider

v. a managed care plan that pays a certain amount to a provider over a specific time for caring for the patients in the plan, regardless of what or how many services are performed

w. the basis of a physician's fee schedule for the normal cost of the same service or procedure in a similar geographic area and under the same or similar circumstances

x. the agreed-upon amount paid to the provider by a policyholder

y. an analysis of individual cases by a committee to make sure services and procedures being billed to a third-party payer are medically necessary

z. the amount paid by the patient before the carrier begins paying

COG SHORT ANSWER

Grade: _____

48. What does the acronym DRG represent? How are DRGs used?

_____

_____

_____

49. What does the acronym RBRVS represent? Briefly explain RBRVS.

50. What is a third-party payer?

51. Elaine is 22 years old and is still eligible as a dependent. What could be a possible reason for this?

52. Why do managed care programs require approved referrals?

53. What does a gatekeeper physician do?

54. A new patient comes to your office, and he hands you his insurance card. What information can you find on the back of his identification card?

55. What form do you fill out to submit an insurance claim?

______

______

______

56. When is a physician required to file a patient's claim or to extend credit?

______

______

______

57. Why is it important to check the Explanation of Benefits?

______

______

______

58. What is a preexisting condition?

______

______

______

COG PSY ACTIVE LEARNING

Grade: ______

59. Interview three people about their health insurance. Ask them what they like about their service. What do they dislike? Compile a list of their comments to discuss with the class.

60. Visit the Web site for Medicare at http://www.medicare.gov. Locate their Frequently Asked Questions page. Read over the questions, and choose five that you believe are the most likely to be asked in a medical office. Design a pamphlet for your office that addresses these five questions.

61. Although a large percentage of Americans have some sort of health insurance, there are still many people who go without. Research online and in medical journals to see what solutions the government and health care companies are devising to reduce the number of uninsured Americans, and to provide better, cheaper, and more widespread health care. Choose one solution, and write a letter to the editor of a local newspaper explaining your position.

COG IDENTIFICATION

Grade: ________

62. Jim works for a company that offers an employee benefit whereby money is taken out of his paycheck and put toward medical care expenses. What is the name of this practice?

____

____

63. Determine which of the following are characteristics of Medicare or Medicaid. Place a check mark in the appropriate column below.

	Medicare	**Medicaid**
a. Provides coverage for low-income or indigent persons of all ages		
b. In a crossover claim, this is the primary coverage		
c. Implemented on a state or local level		
d. Physician reimbursement is considerably less than other insurances		
e. Patients receive a new ID card each month		
f. Program is broken down into part A and part B		
g. Provides coverage for persons suffering from end-stage renal disease		

64. Read each person's health insurance scenario and then match it with the correct type of health insurance plan.

Scenario

a. Sandra was recently let go from her job and is unemployed. _____

b. Thomas has a plan that has less generous coverage and may limit or eliminate benefits for certain illnesses or injuries. _____

c. Mario just started a new job and signed up for health insurance at work. _____

Health Insurance Plan

1. group

2. individual health

3. government

PSY WHAT WOULD YOU DO?

Grade: ______

65. Claims are sometimes denied, and it is your responsibility to take corrective actions. Read the scenarios below, and briefly state what action you should take.

a. Services are not covered by the plan.______

b. Coding is deemed inappropriate for services provided.______

c. Data is incomplete.______

d. Patient cannot be identified as a covered person.______

e. The patient is no longer covered by the plan.______

66. Kairi is a dependent, and both of her parents have health care plans. There are no specific instructions about which plan is primary, so how do you choose which plan to use?

______

______

______

______

67. Describe the two main characteristics of primary and secondary insurance below.

Primary Insurance	Secondary Insurance

COG TRUE OR FALSE?

Grade: ________

68. Determine if the statements below are true or false. If false, explain why.

a. Approximately 80% of Americans are enrolled in health benefits plans of one sort or another.

____

b. A network of providers that make up the PHO may have no financial obligation to subscribers.

____

c. In managed care, a patient is not usually required to use network providers to receive full coverage.

____

d. An HMO requires the patient to pay the provider directly, then reimburses the patient.

____

PSY WHAT WOULD YOU DO?

Grade: ________

69. Mrs. Smith is moving out of the area and is seeing Dr. Jones, her primary care physician, for the last time. After the move, Mrs. Smith will have to choose a new physician. Mrs. Smith has the choice of an HMO or a PPO. Mrs. Smith asks you to explain the difference. How would you teach Mrs. Smith about the differences between an HMO and a PPO?

____

____

____

____

70. Mandy's primary care physician is included under her health plan. However, she has recently been experiencing chest pains, and her physician refers her to a cardiologist. What would you to do to help make sure the specialist's visit is covered?

____

____

____

____

AFF CASE STUDY FOR CRITICAL THINKING

Grade: ________

You are tasked with arranging a referral for Mrs. Williams. She has Blue Cross Blue Shield of VA. She needs a carpal tunnel release. She insists that her insurance will pay, but when you call for preauthorization, you are told her policy is no longer in effect. She did not pay her premium last month, and the policy was cancelled. Apparently she has not been notified.

71. Word for word, what would you say to her?

____

____

____

____

72. Circle all appropriate contacts below that you could suggest to Mrs. Williams.

a. The Yellow Pages

b. The local Department of Social Services

c. An attorney

d. Another physician. She probably will not be able to pay.

e. A free clinic

f. Her employer

g. The phone number on the back of her insurance card

PSY PROCEDURE 13-1 Completing a CMS-1500 Claim Form

Name: ______________________ Date: __________ Time: __________ Grade: __________

EQUIPMENT: Case scenario (see work product), completed encounter form, blank CMS-1500 Claim Form, pen

STANDARDS: Given the needed equipment and a place to work the student will perform this skill with _______% accuracy in a total of _______ minutes. *(Your instructor will tell you what the percentage and time limits will be before you begin.)*

KEY: 4 = Satisfactory 0 = Unsatisfactory NA = This step is not counted

PROCEDURE STEPS	SELF	PARTNER	INSTRUCTOR
1. Using the information provided in the case scenario, complete the demographic information in lines 1 through 11d.	☐	☐	☐
2. Insert "SOF" (signature on file) on lines 12 and 13. Check to be sure there is a current signature on file in the chart and that it is specifically for the third-party payer being filed.	☐	☐	☐
3. If the services being filed are for a hospital stay, insert information in lines 16, 18, and 32.	☐	☐	☐
4. If the services are related to an injury, insert the date of the accident in line 14.	☐	☐	☐
5. Insert dates of service.	☐	☐	☐
6. Using the encounter form, place the CPT code listed for each service and procedure checked off in column D of lines 21–24 on the form.	☐	☐	☐
7. Place the diagnostic codes indicated on the encounter form in lines 21 (1–4). List the reason for the encounter on line 21.1 and any other diagnoses listed on the encounter form that relate to the services or procedures.	☐	☐	☐
8. Reference the codes placed in lines 21 (1–4) to each line listing a different CPT code by placing the corresponding one-digit in line 24, column e.	☐	☐	☐
9. AFF You notice that Mr. Dishman has no signature on file, but the box on line 12 of his claim form says he does. Explain how you would respond.	☐	☐	☐

____

____

____

____

CALCULATION

Total Possible Points: ______

Total Points Earned: ______ Multiplied by 100 = ______ Divided by Total Possible Points = ______ %

PASS ☐ **FAIL** ☐ **COMMENTS:**

Student's signature ______________________ Date ______

Partner's signature ______________________ Date ______

Instructor's signature ______________________ Date ______

WORK PRODUCT 1

Grade: ________

COMPLETE INSURANCE CLAIM FORMS

Jackson Dishman is a 58-year-old man who is seen in the office for acute abdominal pain. Complete the CMS-1500 form using the information provided below:

297-01-2222
Jackson W. Dishman Group #68735
123 Smith Avenue
Winston-Salem NC 27103 Date of Birth: 06-01-49

He is charged for an office visit, which carries the CPT code 99213 and costs $150.00. The doctor has the CMA do a radiologic examination, abdomen; complete acute abdomen series (the CPT code 774022); and the charge for the x-rays is $250.00. The x-rays are normal. He pays nothing today. The physician sends Mr. Dishman home with a diagnosis of acute abdominal pain (IDC-9 code is 789.0). He is to return in 2 days unless the pain becomes unbearable.

PLEASE DO NOT STAPLE IN THIS AREA

PICA

HEALTH INSURANCE CLAIM FORM

PICA

CARRIER

1. MEDICARE (Medicare #) MEDICAID (Medicaid #) CHAMPUS (Sponsor's SSN) CHAMPVA (VA File #) GROUP HEALTH PLAN (SSN or ID) FECA BLK LUNG (SSN) OTHER (ID)

1a. INSURED'S I.D. NUMBER (FOR PROGRAM IN ITEM 1)

2. PATIENT'S NAME (Last Name, First Name, Middle Initial)

3. PATIENT'S BIRTH DATE MM DD YY SEX M F

4. INSURED'S NAME (Last Name, First Name, Middle Initial)

5. PATIENT'S ADDRESS (No., Street)

6. PATIENT RELATIONSHIP TO INSURED Self Spouse Child Other

7. INSURED'S ADDRESS (No., Street)

CITY STATE

8. PATIENT STATUS Single Married Other Employed Full-Time Student Part-Time Student

CITY STATE

ZIP CODE TELEPHONE (Include Area Code) ( )

ZIP CODE TELEPHONE (INCLUDE AREA CODE) ( )

9. OTHER INSURED'S NAME (Last Name, First Name, Middle Initial)

10. IS PATIENT'S CONDITION RELATED TO:

11. INSURED'S POLICY GROUP OR FECA NUMBER

a. OTHER INSURED'S POLICY OR GROUP NUMBER

a. EMPLOYMENT? (CURRENT OR PREVIOUS) YES NO

a. INSURED'S DATE OF BIRTH MM DD YY SEX M F

b. OTHER INSURED'S DATE OF BIRTH MM DD YY SEX M F

b. AUTO ACCIDENT? PLACE (State) YES NO

b. EMPLOYER'S NAME OR SCHOOL NAME

c. EMPLOYER'S NAME OR SCHOOL NAME

c. OTHER ACCIDENT? YES NO

c. INSURANCE PLAN NAME OR PROGRAM NAME

d. INSURANCE PLAN NAME OR PROGRAM NAME

10d. RESERVED FOR LOCAL USE

d. IS THERE ANOTHER HEALTH BENEFIT PLAN? YES NO *If yes,* return to and complete item 9 a-d.

READ BACK OF FORM BEFORE COMPLETING & SIGNING THIS FORM.

12. PATIENT'S OR AUTHORIZED PERSON'S SIGNATURE I authorize the release of any medical or other information necessary to process this claim. I also request payment of government benefits either to myself or to the party who accepts assignment below.

SIGNED ______ DATE ______

13. INSURED'S OR AUTHORIZED PERSON'S SIGNATURE I authorize payment of medical benefits to the undersigned physician or supplier for services described below.

SIGNED ______

PATIENT AND INSURED INFORMATION

14. DATE OF CURRENT: MM DD YY ◄ ILLNESS (First symptom) OR INJURY (Accident) OR PREGNANCY(LMP)

15. IF PATIENT HAS HAD SAME OR SIMILAR ILLNESS. GIVE FIRST DATE MM DD YY

16. DATES PATIENT UNABLE TO WORK IN CURRENT OCCUPATION FROM MM DD YY TO MM DD YY

17. NAME OF REFERRING PHYSICIAN OR OTHER SOURCE

17a. I.D. NUMBER OF REFERRING PHYSICIAN

18. HOSPITALIZATION DATES RELATED TO CURRENT SERVICES FROM MM DD YY TO MM DD YY

19. RESERVED FOR LOCAL USE

20. OUTSIDE LAB? YES NO $ CHARGES

21. DIAGNOSIS OR NATURE OF ILLNESS OR INJURY. (RELATE ITEMS 1,2,3 OR 4 TO ITEM 24E BY LINE)

1. ___ . __
2. ___ . __
3. ___ . __
4. ___ . __

22. MEDICAID RESUBMISSION CODE ORIGINAL REF. NO.

23. PRIOR AUTHORIZATION NUMBER

24. A DATE(S) OF SERVICE From MM DD YY To MM DD YY	B Place of Service	C Type of Service	D PROCEDURES, SERVICES, OR SUPPLIES (Explain Unusual Circumstances) CPT/HCPCS MODIFIER	E DIAGNOSIS CODE	F $ CHARGES	G DAYS OR UNITS	H EPSDT Family Plan	I EMG	J COB	K RESERVED FOR LOCAL USE
1										
2										
3										
4										
5										
6										

25. FEDERAL TAX I.D. NUMBER SSN EIN

26. PATIENT'S ACCOUNT NO.

27. ACCEPT ASSIGNMENT? (For govt. claims, see back) YES NO

28. TOTAL CHARGE $

29. AMOUNT PAID $

30. BALANCE DUE $

31. SIGNATURE OF PHYSICIAN OR SUPPLIER INCLUDING DEGREES OR CREDENTIALS (I certify that the statements on the reverse apply to this bill and are made a part thereof.)

SIGNED DATE

32. NAME AND ADDRESS OF FACILITY WHERE SERVICES WERE RENDERED (If other than home or office)

33. PHYSICIAN'S, SUPPLIER'S BILLING NAME, ADDRESS, ZIP CODE & PHONE #

PIN# GRP#

PHYSICIAN OR SUPPLIER INFORMATION

(APPROVED BY AMA COUNCIL ON MEDICAL SERVICE 8/88) ***PLEASE PRINT OR TYPE*** APPROVED OMB-0938-0008 FORM CMS-1500 (12-90), FORM RRB-1500, APPROVED OMB-1215-0055 FORM OWCP-1500, APPROVED OMB-0720-0001 (CHAMPUS)

CHAPTER

14 Diagnostic Coding

Learning Outcomes

Cognitive Domain

1. Spell and define the key terms
2. Describe the relationship between coding and reimbursement
3. Name and describe the coding system used to describe diseases, injuries, and other reasons for encounters with a medical provider
4. Explain the format of the ICD-9-CM
5. Give four examples of ways E codes are used
6. Describe how to use the most current diagnostic coding classification system
7. Describe the ICD-10-CM/PCS version and its differences from ICD-9

Psychomotor Domain

1. Perform diagnostic coding (Procedure 14-1)
2. Apply third-party guidelines

Affective Domain

1. Work with physician to achieve the maximum reimbursement

ABHES Competencies

1. Apply third-party guidelines
2. Perform diagnostic and procedural coding
3. Comply with federal, state, and local health laws and regulations

Name: ______________________ Date: __________ Grade: __________

COG MULTIPLE CHOICE

1. Which most accurately states the purpose of coding?
   - a. Coding assists patients in accessing insurance databases.
   - b. Coding determines the reimbursement of medical fees.
   - c. Coding is used to track a physician's payments.
   - d. Coding is used to index patients' claims forms.
   - e. Coding identifies patients in a database.
2. A patient signs an advance beneficiary notice (ABN) to:
   - a. consent to medically necessary procedures.
   - b. assign payment to Medicare.
   - c. accept responsibility for payment.
   - d. assign responsibility for payment to a beneficiary.
   - e. consent to a medically unnecessary procedure.
3. The content of the ICD-9-CM is a(n):
   - a. classification of diseases and list of procedures.
   - b. statistical grouping of trends in diseases.
   - c. clinical modification of codes used by hospitals.
   - d. ninth volume in an index of diseases.
   - e. international document for monitoring coding.
4. Which is true of Volume 3 of the ICD-9-CM?
   - a. It is organized by location on the patient's body.
   - b. It is used to code mostly outpatient procedures.
   - c. It is an alphabetical listing of diseases.
   - d. It is used by hospitals to report procedures and services.
   - e. It is an index of Volumes 1 and 2.
5. Physicians' services are reported:
   - a. on the UB-04.
   - b. on the CMS-1500.
   - c. on the uniform bill.
   - d. on the advance beneficiary notice.
   - e. on bills from health institutions.
6. Which of these would be considered inpatient coding?
   - a. Hospital same-day surgery
   - b. Hour-long testing in a hospital CAT scan
   - c. Treatment in the emergency room
   - d. Observation status in a hospital
   - e. Meals and testing during a hospital stay
7. In Volume 1 of the ICD-9-CM, chapters are grouped:
   - a. by alphabetic ordering of diseases and injuries.
   - b. alphabetically by eponym.
   - c. by location in the body.
   - d. by etiology and anatomic system.
   - e. by surgical specialty.
8. The fourth and fifth digits in a code indicate the:
   - a. anatomical location where a procedure was performed.
   - b. number of times a test was executed.
   - c. higher definitions of a code.
   - d. code for the patient's general disease.
   - e. traumatic origins of a disease (i.e., injury, deliberate violence).
9. A V-code might indicate a(n):
   - a. immunization.
   - b. poisoning.
   - c. accident.
   - d. diagnosis.
   - e. treatment.
10. V-codes are used:
    - a. for outpatient coding.
    - b. when reimbursement is not needed.
    - c. when a patient is not sick.
    - d. to indicate testing for HIV.
    - e. for infectious diseases.

11. What is the purpose of E-codes?

a. They code for immunizations and other preventive procedures.

b. They are used to code medical testing before a diagnosis.

c. They assist insurance companies in making reimbursements.

d. They indicate why a patient has an injury or poisoning.

e. They indicate if a procedure was inpatient or outpatient.

12. Which of the following agencies are least interested in E-codes?

a. Insurance underwriters

b. Insurance claim providers

c. National safety programs

d. Public health agencies

e. Workers' compensation lawyers

13. How is Volume 2 of the ICD-9-CM different from Volume 1?

a. Volume 2 contains diagnostic terms that are not used in Volume 1.

b. Volume 2 is organized into 17 chapters rather than 3 sections.

c. Volume 2 does not contain E-codes, but Volume 1 does.

d. Volume 2 contains hospital coding to cross-reference with Volume 1.

e. Volume 2 provides information about the fourth and fifth digits of a code.

14. After finding a code in Volume 2, you should:

a. record the code on the CMS-1500.

b. consult Volume 3 for subordinate terms.

c. cross-reference the code with Volume 1.

d. indicate if the code is inpatient or outpatient.

e. record the code on the UB-04.

15. Volume 3 of the ICD-9-CM is organized:

a. by disease.

b. by anatomy.

c. into 17 chapters.

d. into three sections.

e. by surgical specialty.

16. One example of an eponym is:

a. Crohn disease.

b. bacterial meningitis.

c. influenza virus.

d. pruritus.

e. pneumonia.

17. What is the first step to locating a diagnostic code?

a. Determine where the diagnosis occurs in the body.

b. Choose the main term within the diagnostic statement.

c. Begin looking up the diagnosis in Volume 1 of the ICD-9-CM.

d. Consult the CMS-1500 for reimbursement codes.

e. Use Volume 3 of the ICD-9-CM to find the disease.

18. Which code is listed first on a CMS-1500?

a. A reasonable second opinion

b. Relevant laboratory work

c. Diagnostic tests

d. The symptoms of an illness

e. The primary diagnosis

19. How do you code for late effects?

a. Code for the treatment of the disease that causes late effects.

b. Code for the disease that is causing the current condition.

c. First code for the current condition, and then list the cause.

d. Only code for the current condition.

e. Only code for the cause of the current condition.

20. You should not code for a brain tumor:

a. when the patient comes in for an MRI.

b. after the tumor is confirmed on an MRI.

c. when the diagnosed patient comes in for treatment.

d. any time after the patient has been diagnosed.

e. when the patient seeks specialist care.

COG MATCHING

Grade: _____

Match the following key terms to their definitions.

Key Terms

21. _____ advance beneficiary notice

22. _____ audits

23. _____ conventions

24. _____ cross-reference

25. _____ E-codes

26. _____ eponym

27. _____ etiology

28. _____ inpatient

29. _____ International Classification of Diseases, Ninth Revision, Clinical Modification

30. _____ late effects

31. _____ main terms

32. _____ medical necessity

33. _____ outpatient

34. _____ primary diagnosis

35. _____ service

36. _____ specificity

37. _____ V-codes

Definitions

a. codes indicating the external causes of injuries and poisoning

b. conditions that result from another condition

c. general notes, symbols, typeface, format, and punctuation that direct and guide a coder to the most accurate ICD-9 code

d. the condition or chief complaint that brings a person to a medical facility for treatment

e. a procedure or service that would have been performed by any reasonable physician under the same or similar circumstances

f. a document that informs covered patients that Medicare may not cover a certain service and the patient will be responsible for the bill

g. a word based on or derived from a person's name

h. codes assigned to patients who receive service but have no illness, injury, or disorder

i. the billable tasks performed by a physician

j. refers to a medical setting in which patients are admitted for diagnostic, radiographic, or treatment purposes

k. an investigation performed by government, managed health care companies, and health care organizations to determine compliance and to detect fraud

l. a system for transforming verbal descriptions of disease, injuries, conditions, and procedures to numeric codes

m. refers to the cause of disease

n. refers to a medical setting in which patients receive care but are not admitted

o. verification against another source

p. relating to a definite result

q. words in a multiple-word diagnosis that a coder should locate in the alphabetic listing

COG SHORT ANSWER

Grade: ________

38. Why is the third volume of the ICD-9-CM not used at a hospital's emergency department?

39. What is the title of the new edition of the ICD manuals? When will the new codes go into effect?

40. You are reading a patient's chart and notice that it is marked with an E-code. However, the patient has experienced no physical injuries. Why might an E-code be used in this situation?

41. You ask a veteran medical assistant for advice on coding, especially how to go about finding a diagnosis with more than one word. Her response is, "Find the condition, not the location." What does she mean by this?

42. What is listed first in the diagnosis section of the CMS-1500? What does it represent?

43. If a construction worker falls from a ladder and suffers an ankle fracture, what supplemental code is used?

44. When would you use the V-code for laboratory examination?

45. What should you do after finding a seemingly appropriate code in the alphabetic listing of Volume 1 of the ICD-9-CM?

46. If you do not know the medical terminology for a diagnosis for a common problem, what would be a good first plan of action?

47. What is the purpose of the fourth and fifth digits often appended to categories?

COG PSY **ACTIVE LEARNING** Grade: ________

48. A reasonable and capable physician believes that a patient needs a chest x-ray to rule out pneumonia. Does the procedure meet the grounds for medical necessity? Why? Why not?

49. A patient comes in complaining of chest pain. When you enter the codes for this patient encounter, you code that the patient has "acute myocardial infarction." Why would it be better to code this encounter "chest pain rule out myocardial infarction"?

50. George Cregan has been seen by the physician for controlled non–insulin-dependent type 2 diabetes mellitus for about 10 years. While being seen for a routine check of his blood sugar, he complains of numbness and tingling in his left lower leg and foot. An x-ray of both legs is performed because poor circulation in the extremities can be a complication of diabetes. The x-ray confirms the diagnosis of peripheral neuropathy. Which ICD-9 code should be listed with the office visit? Which code indicates the reason for the x-ray? Which code should be placed on the CMA-1500 first as the primary diagnosis or reason for the visit?

51. In the ICD-9-CM, burns are listed in the range 940–949, a subset of 800–999—Injury and Poisoning. However, if you look for the code for sunburn, you will not find it there. Find the code for sunburn and explain why it does not belong in the range 940–949. You do not need to know exactly why, but consider the diagnoses that appear in 940–949 and how sunburn compares with them.

____

____

____

____

Determine the main term for the following multiple-word diagnoses.

Diagnosis	Main Term
52. chronic fatigue syndrome	
53. severe acute respiratory syndrome	
54. hemorrhagic encephalitis	
55. acute fulminating multiple sclerosis	
56. fractured left tibia	
57. breast cyst	

COG IDENTIFICATION

Grade: _______

58. Review the list of circumstances below and place a check mark to indicate whether a patient would be forced, given the circumstance, to sign an ABN. All of the patients below are covered by Medicare.

Circumstance	ABN	No ABN
a. The patient wishes to receive an immunization not covered by Medicare.		
b. The patient is undergoing a regularly scheduled checkup.		
c. The patient demands to be tested for an illness that the physician considers an impossibility.		
d. The patient has a badly sprained ankle and wishes to be treated.		
e. The patient is undergoing x-ray imaging per order of a physician.		

59. When it comes to coding, it makes a difference if the patient is seen in an inpatient or outpatient facility. Review the list of places below. Place an ***I*** next to those places that are considered "Inpatient" and an ***O*** next to those places that are considered "Outpatient."

a. ______ Hospital clinic

b. ______ Health care provider's office

c. ______ Hospital for less than 24 hours

d. ______ Hospital for 24 hours or more

e. ______ Hospital emergency room

60. Circle the main terms where you will find obstetric conditions.

delivery	fetus	pregnancy	labor
baby	obstetrics	puerperal	gestational

COG TRUE OR FALSE?

Grade: ______

True or False? Determine whether the following statements are true or false. If false, explain why.

61. Only the first three numbers of a code are necessary.

____

62. One should never code directly from the alphabetic index.

____

63. The main term describes a condition, not an aspect of anatomy.

____

64. In the outpatient setting, coders list conditions after the patient's testing is complete.

____

AFF WHAT WOULD YOU DO?

Grade: ______

65. A patient calls complaining of pain and swelling in the right hand since awakening this morning. The patient comes in, sees the doctor, and returns to the front desk with an encounter form that states his diagnosis is "gout." In order to make this diagnosis, the physician would need to know the patient's uric acid level. You know that the patient just had blood drawn for the test. It is a test that must be sent to an outside lab. Do you still code today's visit as "gout"? What would you do?

____

____

____

____

66. A patient is concerned that her insurance provider will not cover her visit because the diagnosis is for a very minor ailment. She requests that you mark her CMA-1500 with a more severe disorder that demands similar treatment. How would you deal with this situation? What would you tell the patient? How might you involve the physician?

67. A patient entered the office complaining of chest pains. After examination, the physician decided to send him to a specialist in order to rule out the possibility of angina pectoris. Which code should be placed on the CMA-1500 first as the primary diagnosis or reason for the visit? Why?

AFF CASE STUDY FOR CRITICAL THINKING

Grade: ______

Your physician-employer works with you closely to choose the most appropriate codes. He tells you that he would like for you to code patients who have B_{12} injections with "pernicious anemia." You ask if these patients should have a lab work to substantiate that diagnosis, and he says, "don't worry about that."

68. What would you say to him?

69. What would be the possible consequences of such an action?

70. Which of these is an unethical act? Explain why.

a. Coding multiple conditions on the same CMS-1500

b. Coding an unsupported diagnosis in order to make a service appear medically necessary

c. Using a V-code to better explain the reason for a patient's visit

d. Using ICD-9-CM search software to more easily access the codes contained in the ICD-9-CM

PSY PROCEDURE 14-1 Locating a Diagnostic Code

Name: ______________________ Date: __________ Time: __________ Grade: __________

EQUIPMENT: Diagnosis, ICD-9-CM, Volumes 1 and 2 codebook, medical dictionary.

STANDARDS: Given the needed equipment and a place to work the student will perform this skill with ________% accuracy in a total of ________ minutes. *(Your instructor will tell you what the percentage and time limits will be before you begin.)*

KEY: 4 = Satisfactory 0 = Unsatisfactory NA = this step is not counted

PROCEDURE STEPS	SELF	PARTNER	INSTRUCTOR
1. Using the diagnosis "chronic rheumatoid arthritis," choose the main term within the diagnostic statement. If necessary, look up the word(s) in your dictionary.	☐	☐	☐
2. Locate the main term in Volume 2.	☐	☐	☐
3. Refer to all notes and conventions under the main term.	☐	☐	☐
4. Find the appropriate indented subordinate term.	☐	☐	☐
5. Follow any relevant instructions, such as "see also."	☐	☐	☐
6. Confirm the selected code by cross-referencing to Volume 1. Make sure you have added any fourth or fifth digits necessary.	☐	☐	☐
7. Assign the code.	☐	☐	☐
8. AFF Your office manager instructs you to assign a diagnosis code to a claim for a patient that you know does not have the diagnosis. Explain how you would respond.	☐	☐	☐

____

____

____

____

CALCULATION

Total Possible Points: ______

Total Points Earned: ________ Multiplied by 100 = ________ Divided by Total Possible Points = ________ %

PASS ☐ **FAIL** ☐ **COMMENTS:**

Student's signature ______________________ Date ______

Partner's signature ______________________ Date ______

Instructor's signature ______________________ Date ______

WORK PRODUCT 1

Grade: ________

Underline the main term in these diagnoses with more than one word. Using a current ICD-9-CM book, then code the diagnoses:

1. sick sinus syndrome
2. congestive heart failure with malignant hypertension
3. bilateral stenosis of carotid artery
4. aspiration pneumonia
5. massive blood transfusion thrombocytopenia
6. acute rheumatic endocarditis
7. acute viral conjunctivitis with hemorrhage
8. *E. coli* intestinal infection
9. postgastrectomy diarrhea
10. congenital syphilitic osteomyelitis

WORK PRODUCT 2

Grade: ________

Determine the diseases associated with the following ICD-9-CM codes:

1. 555.9

____

2. 676.54

____

3. 314.01

____

4. 726.71

____

5. 722.93

____

WORK PRODUCT 3

Grade: ______

Determine the E-codes for the following:

1. Injured when hot air balloon crashed

____

2. Skin frozen, contact with dry ice

____

3. Bicyclist injured by train

____

4. Injured by fireworks

____

5. Hand slashed by circular saw

____

WORK PRODUCT 4

Grade: ______

Code Sequencing

Kayla Moore, age 38 years, is seen in the clinic today. She has a few chronic conditions but is seen today for fluttering in her chest. Because she is here, and it is time for her regular diabetes checkup, the doctor orders a test to check on her blood sugar. Because Ms. Moore is a breast cancer survivor, in addition she was given a mammogram. Her physician also prescribed a tetanus booster as well, because she has been renovating an old stable and has suffered several small skin punctures over the past few weeks. Her encounter form indicates the following charges:

- an EKG to monitor a previously diagnosed arrhythmia
- fasting blood sugar for known diabetes
- mammogram
- tetanus booster

List the diagnoses in the proper order to be placed on line #21 of the CMS-1500 form.

21.

1.______________ 3.______________

2.______________ 4.______________

CHAPTER

15 Outpatient Procedural Coding

Learning Outcomes

Cognitive Domain

1. Spell and define the key terms
2. Explain the Healthcare Common Procedure Coding System (HCPCS), levels I and II
3. Explain the format of level I, Current Procedural Terminology (CPT-4) and its use
4. Describe the relationship between coding and reimbursement
5. Describe how to use the most current procedure coding system
6. Define upcoding and why it should be avoided
7. Describe how to uses the most current HCPCS coding
8. Describe the concept of RBRVS
9. Discuss all levels of governmental legislation and regulation as they apply to medical assisting practice, including FDA and DEA regulations
10. Define both medical terms and abbreviations related to all body systems

Psychomotor Domain

1. Perform procedural coding (Procedure 15-1)
2. Apply third-party guidelines

Affective Domain

1. Work with physician to achieve the maximum reimbursement
2. Demonstrate assertive communication with managed care and/or insurance providers
3. Apply ethical behaviors, including honesty/integrity in performance of medical assisting practice

ABHES Competencies

1. Apply third-party guidelines
2. Perform diagnostic and procedural coding
3. Comply with federal, state, and local health laws and regulations

Name: ______________________ Date: ____________ Grade: ____________

COG MULTIPLE CHOICE

1. In the case of an unlisted code, the medical assistant should:
   - a. notify the AMA so that a new code is issued.
   - b. submit a copy of the procedure report with the claim.
   - c. obtain authorization from the AMA to proceed with the procedure.
   - d. include the code that fits the most and add a note to explain the differences.
   - e. not charge the patient for the procedure.

2. Which kind of information appears in a special report?
   - a. Type of medicine prescribed
   - b. Patient history
   - c. Allergic reactions
   - d. Possible procedural risks
   - e. Equipment necessary for the treatment

3. On a medical record, the key components contained in E/M codes indicate:
   - a. the scope and result of a medical visit.
   - b. the duties of a physician toward his patients.
   - c. the definition and description of a performed procedure.
   - d. the services that a medical assistant may perform.
   - e. the charges that are owed to the insurance company.

4. Time becomes a key component in a medical record when:
   - a. the visit lasts more than 1 hour.
   - b. more than half of the visit is spent counseling.
   - c. the physician decides for a series of regular visits.
   - d. the visit lasts longer than it was initially established.
   - e. the patient is constantly late for his or her appointments.

5. When assigning a level of medical decision making, you should consider the:
   - a. medication the patient is on.
   - b. available coding for the procedure.
   - c. patient's symptoms during the visit.
   - d. insurance coverage allowed to the patient.
   - e. patient's medical history.

6. In the anesthesia section, the physical status modifier indicates the patient's:
   - a. medical history.
   - b. conditions after surgery.
   - c. good health before surgery.
   - d. reactions to past anesthesia.
   - e. condition prior to the administration of anesthesia.

7. Which of the following is included in a surgical package?
   - a. General anesthesia
   - b. Hospitalization time
   - c. Complications related to the surgery
   - d. Prescriptions given after the operation
   - e. Uncomplicated follow-up care

8. How are procedures organized in the subsections of the surgery section of the CPT-4?
   - a. By invasiveness
   - b. By location and type
   - c. In alphabetical order
   - d. In order of difficulty of procedure
   - e. By average recurrence of procedure

9. Which is the first digit that appears on radiology codes?
   - a. 1
   - b. 6
   - c. 7
   - d. 8
   - e. 9

10. Diagnostic-related groups (DRGs) are a group of:

a. codes pertaining to one particular treatment.

b. inpatients sharing a similar medical history.

c. modifiers attached to a single procedural form.

d. physicians agreeing on a procedure for a particular medical condition.

e. inpatients sharing similar diagnoses, treatment, and length of hospital stay.

11. The resource-based relative value scale (RBRVS) gives information on the:

a. difficulty level of a particular surgical operation.

b. maximum fee that physicians can charge for a procedure.

c. reimbursement given to physicians for Medicare services.

d. average fee asked by physicians for emergency procedures.

e. minimum amount of time the physician should spend with a patient.

12. The Medicare allowed charge is calculated by:

a. adding the RVU and the national conversion factor.

b. dividing the RVU by the national conversion factor.

c. multiplying the RVU by the national conversion factor.

d. subtracting the RVU from the national conversion factor.

e. finding the average between the RVU and the national conversion factor.

13. Upcoding is:

a. billing more than the proper fee for a service.

b. correcting an erroneous code in medical records.

c. auditing claims retroactively for suspected fraud.

d. comparing the documentation in the record with the codes received.

e. researching new codes online.

14. Who has jurisdiction over a fraudulent medical practice?

a. CMS

b. AMA

c. Medicare

d. U.S. Attorney General

e. State's supreme court

15. The purpose of the Level II HCPCS codes is to:

a. decode different types of code modifiers.

b. attribute a code to every step of a medical procedure.

c. list the practices eligible for reimbursement by Medicare.

d. identify services, supplies, and equipment not identified by CPT codes.

e. provide coding information for various types of anesthesia.

16. Which of these sections is included in the HCPCS Level I code listing?

a. Orthotics

b. Injections

c. Vision care

d. Dental services

e. Pathology and laboratory

17. How is a consultation different from a referral?

a. A consultation is needed when the patient wants to change physicians.

b. A consultation is needed when the physician asks for the opinion of another provider.

c. A consultation is needed when the patient is transferred to another physician for treatment.

d. A consultation is needed when the physician needs a team of doctors to carry out a procedure.

e. A consultation is needed before the physician can submit insurance claims.

18. Which of the following is contained in Appendix B in the CPT-4?

a. Legislation against medical fraud

b. Detailed explanation of the modifiers

c. Revisions made since the last editions

d. Explanation on how to file for reimbursement

e. Examples concerning the Evaluation and Management sections

19. Drug screening is considered *quantitative* when checking:

- **a.** for the amount of illegal drugs in the blood.
- **b.** for the presence of illegal drugs in the blood.
- **c.** for the proper level of therapeutic drugs in the blood.
- **d.** that the therapeutic drug is not interacting with other medications.
- **e.** that the drug is not causing an allergic reaction.

20. Which place requires the use of an emergency department service code?

- **a.** Private clinic
- **b.** Nursing home
- **c.** Physician's office
- **d.** 24-hour pharmacy
- **e.** Mental health center

21. How many numbers do E/M codes have?

- **a.** Two
- **b.** Five
- **c.** Six
- **d.** Seven
- **e.** Ten

COG MATCHING

Grade: _____

Match the following key terms to their definitions.

Key Terms

22. _____ Current Procedural Terminology

23. _____ descriptor

24. _____ diagnostic-related group

25. _____ Health Care Common Procedure Coding System

26. _____ key component

27. _____ modifiers

28. _____ outlier

29. _____ procedure

30. _____ resource-based relative value scale

31. _____ upcoding

Definitions

- **a.** a patient whose hospital stay is longer than amount allowed by the DRG
- **b.** categories used to determine hospital and physician reimbursement for Medicare patients' inpatient services
- **c.** a value scale designed to decrease Medicare Part B costs and establish national standards for coding and payment
- **d.** billing more than the proper fee for a service by selecting a code that is higher on the coding scale
- **e.** description of a service listed with its code number
- **f.** numbers or letters added to a code to clarify the service or procedure provided
- **g.** a comprehensive listing of medical terms and codes for the uniform coding of procedures and services that are provided by physicians
- **h.** a medical service or test that is coded for reimbursement
- **i.** a standardized coding system that is used primarily to identify products, supplies, and services
- **j.** the criteria or factors on which the selection of CPT-4 evaluation and management is based

COG SHORT ANSWER

Grade: ________

32. What role do modifiers play in coding?

33. When would you use 99 as the first numbers in your modifier?

34. What is the goal of the RBRVS?

35. How does coding play a part in reimbursement?

36. What are DRGs, and how are they used to determine Medicare payments?

37. List three ways to reduce the likelihood of a Medicare audit of your office.

38. Name four factors that go into radiology coding.

39. Why is it important to check the components of a surgery package with a third-party payer?

40. A patient experiences complications after an appendectomy and has to be hospitalized for several days. Will the time spent in the hospital be coded as part of a surgery package or separately?

COG PSY ACTIVE LEARNING

Grade: ______

Using a current CPT book, assign the appropriate CPT code for the following:

41. occult blood in stool, two simultaneous guaiac tests

____

42. blood ethanol levels

____

43. transurethral resection of prostate

____

44. flexible sigmoidoscopy for biopsy

____

45. radiation therapy requiring general anesthesia

____

46. hair transplant, 21 punch grafts

____

47. breast reduction, left

____

48. open repair of left Dupuytren contracture

____

49. partial removal left turbinate

____

50. newborn clamp circumcision

____

COG PSY IDENTIFICATION

Grade: ________

What digit would be the first digit of the following codes?

51. routine prothrombin time

52. ultrasound guidance for amniocentesis

53. well-child check

54. EKG

55. removal of skin tags

COG TRUE OR FALSE?

Grade: ________

Determine whether the following statements are true or false. If false, explain why.

56. It is permissible to leave out modifiers if a note is made on the patient's sheet.

57. When time spent with a patient is more than 50% of the typical time for the visit, time becomes the deciding factor in choosing a code.

58. The number of tests you perform is the final number in the coding.

59. The amount of time a physician spends with a patient has no effect on the coding for that exam.

COG IDENTIFICATION

Grade: __________

60. Fill in the chart below to show the difference between Level I HPCS and Level II.

Level I	Level II

61. What are the six major sections of the CPT-4?

a. ____

b. ____

c. ____

d. ____

e. ____

f. ____

62. Define the seven components of the E/M codes.

Component	Definition
a. history	
b. physician examination	
c. medical decision making	
d. counseling	
e. coordination of care	
f. nature of presenting problem	
g. time	

PSY WHAT WOULD YOU DO?

Grade: ________

63. Read the scenario below. Then, highlight or underline the medical decision-making section.
Anikka was seen today for a followup on her broken wrist. The cast was removed 2 weeks ago, and she said she is still unable to achieve full range of movement in her wrist without pain. On exam, her wrist appeared swollen, and she mentioned tenderness. X-ray revealed slight fracture in carpals. Dr. Levy splinted the wrist, and referred her to an orthopedic surgeon for possible surgery. I spoke with Anikka, instructing her to avoid exerting her wrist and to keep it splinted until she has seen the surgeon. Dr. Levy suggested aspirin for pain.

64. Now, read the same scenario again. Circle the history section.
Anikka was seen today for a followup on her broken wrist. The cast was removed 2 weeks ago, and she said she is still unable to achieve full range of movement in her wrist without pain. On exam, her wrist appeared swollen, and she mentioned tenderness. X-ray revealed slight fracture in carpals. Dr. Levy splinted the wrist, and referred her to an orthopedic surgeon for possible surgery. I spoke with Anikka, instructing her to avoid exerting her wrist and to keep it splinted until she has seen the surgeon. Dr. Levy suggested aspirin for pain.

65. Read the scenario below.
Mr. Ekko presents today for removal of stitches from calf wound. Upon inspection, wound seems to have healed well, but scar tissue is still slightly inflamed. I prescribed antibacterial cream for him to apply twice a day, and instructed him to still keep the area bandaged. I told him to let us know if the swelling has not gone down within a week, and to come in if it gets any worse.

Circle the correct level of medical decision making involved.

Straightforward   Low complexity

Moderate complexity   High complexity

COG IDENTIFICATION

Grade: ________

Fill in the medical terminology chart below about the CPT subcategory on repair, revision, or reconstruction.

Suffix	Meaning
66. -pexy	
	67. surgical repair
68. -rrhaphy	

AFF CASE STUDY FOR CRITICAL THINKING

Grade: _______

69. A patient will be undergoing surgery to remove her gallbladder. Her insurance company labels this sort of operation as an outpatient surgery. She lives alone with no assistance after surgery. She wants to stay in the hospital overnight. The patient asks if you can do anything in the coding of the procedure to make her insurance company pay for a night in the hospital. What do you say to her? Can you do anything to code this information on the claim form for more reimbursement?

____

____

____

____

PSY **PROCEDURE 15-1** **Locating a CPT Code**

Name: ______________________________ Date: __________ Time: __________ Grade: __________

EQUIPMENT: CPT-4 codebook, patient chart, scenario (Work Product 1)

STANDARDS Given the needed equipment and a place to work the student will perform this skill with ______% accuracy in a total of ______ minutes. *(Your instructor will tell you what the percentage and time limits will be before you begin.)*

KEY: 4 = Satisfactory 0 = Unsatisfactory NA = This step is not counted

PROCEDURE STEPS	SELF	PARTNER	INSTRUCTOR
1. Identify the exact procedure performed.	☐	☐	☐
2. Obtain the documentation of the procedure in the patient's chart.	☐	☐	☐
3. Choose the proper codebook.	☐	☐	☐
4. Using the alphabetic index, locate the procedure.	☐	☐	☐
5. Locate the code or range of codes given in the tabular section.	☐	☐	☐
6. Read the descriptors to find the one that most closely describes the procedure.	☐	☐	☐
7. Check the section guidelines for any special circumstances.	☐	☐	☐
8. Review the documentation to be sure it justifies the code.	☐	☐	☐
9. Determine if any modifiers are needed.	☐	☐	☐
10. Select the code and place it in the appropriate field of the CMS-1500 form.	☐	☐	☐
11. AFF Your physician is helping you find a code in the CPT-4 codebook. He chooses a code based on what the surgery entailed, but the operative report does not support what he says he did. Explain how you would advise the physician to correct the problem and proceed.	☐	☐	☐

____

____

____

____

CALCULATION

Total Possible Points: ______

Total Points Earned: ______ Multiplied by 100 = ______ Divided by Total Possible Points = ______ %

PASS ☐ **FAIL** ☐ **COMMENTS:**

Student's signature ______________________________ Date ______

Partner's signature ______________________________ Date ______

Instructor's signature ______________________________ Date ______

WORK PRODUCT 1

Grade: _________

Perform Procedural Coding

Kayla Moore, age 38 years, has just completed a general physical. Her examination consisted of the following:

- an EKG to monitor a previously diagnosed arrhythmia
- urine collection to test for diabetes
- blood sampling to test cholesterol levels

Because Ms. Moore is a breast cancer survivor, in addition to the routine examination, she was given a mammogram. Her physician prescribed a tetanus booster as well, because she has been renovating an old stable and has suffered several small skin punctures over the past few weeks.

Complete the CMS-1500 form with the proper procedural coding for the patient's visit. Use the same personal patient information you used for Work Product 1 in Chapter 14 to fill in all essential details when completing the CMS-1500.

PLEASE DO NOT STAPLE IN THIS AREA

PICA

HEALTH INSURANCE CLAIM FORM

PICA

CARRIER

1. MEDICARE (Medicare #) MEDICAID (Medicaid #) CHAMPUS (Sponsor's SSN) CHAMPVA (VA File #) GROUP HEALTH PLAN (SSN or ID) FECA BLK LUNG (SSN) OTHER (ID)

1a. INSURED'S I.D. NUMBER (FOR PROGRAM IN ITEM 1)

2. PATIENT'S NAME (Last Name, First Name, Middle Initial)

3. PATIENT'S BIRTH DATE MM DD YY SEX M F

4. INSURED'S NAME (Last Name, First Name, Middle Initial)

5. PATIENT'S ADDRESS (No., Street)

6. PATIENT RELATIONSHIP TO INSURED Self Spouse Child Other

7. INSURED'S ADDRESS (No., Street)

CITY STATE

8. PATIENT STATUS Single Married Other Employed Full-Time Student Part-Time Student

CITY STATE

ZIP CODE TELEPHONE (Include Area Code) ( )

ZIP CODE TELEPHONE (INCLUDE AREA CODE) ( )

9. OTHER INSURED'S NAME (Last Name, First Name, Middle Initial)

10. IS PATIENT'S CONDITION RELATED TO:

11. INSURED'S POLICY GROUP OR FECA NUMBER

a. OTHER INSURED'S POLICY OR GROUP NUMBER

a. EMPLOYMENT? (CURRENT OR PREVIOUS) YES NO

a. INSURED'S DATE OF BIRTH MM DD YY SEX M F

b. OTHER INSURED'S DATE OF BIRTH MM DD YY SEX M F

b. AUTO ACCIDENT? PLACE (State) YES NO

b. EMPLOYER'S NAME OR SCHOOL NAME

c. EMPLOYER'S NAME OR SCHOOL NAME

c. OTHER ACCIDENT? YES NO

c. INSURANCE PLAN NAME OR PROGRAM NAME

d. INSURANCE PLAN NAME OR PROGRAM NAME

10d. RESERVED FOR LOCAL USE

d. IS THERE ANOTHER HEALTH BENEFIT PLAN? YES NO *If yes,* return to and complete item 9 a-d.

READ BACK OF FORM BEFORE COMPLETING & SIGNING THIS FORM.

12. PATIENT'S OR AUTHORIZED PERSON'S SIGNATURE I authorize the release of any medical or other information necessary to process this claim. I also request payment of government benefits either to myself or to the party who accepts assignment below.

SIGNED ______ DATE ______

13. INSURED'S OR AUTHORIZED PERSON'S SIGNATURE I authorize payment of medical benefits to the undersigned physician or supplier for services described below.

SIGNED ______

PATIENT AND INSURED INFORMATION

14. DATE OF CURRENT: MM DD YY ILLNESS (First symptom) OR INJURY (Accident) OR PREGNANCY(LMP)

15. IF PATIENT HAS HAD SAME OR SIMILAR ILLNESS. GIVE FIRST DATE MM DD YY

16. DATES PATIENT UNABLE TO WORK IN CURRENT OCCUPATION FROM MM DD YY TO MM DD YY

17. NAME OF REFERRING PHYSICIAN OR OTHER SOURCE

17a. I.D. NUMBER OF REFERRING PHYSICIAN

18. HOSPITALIZATION DATES RELATED TO CURRENT SERVICES FROM MM DD YY TO MM DD YY

19. RESERVED FOR LOCAL USE

20. OUTSIDE LAB? YES NO $ CHARGES

21. DIAGNOSIS OR NATURE OF ILLNESS OR INJURY. (RELATE ITEMS 1,2,3 OR 4 TO ITEM 24E BY LINE)

1. ___ . ___ 3. ___ . ___

2. ___ . ___ 4. ___ . ___

22. MEDICAID RESUBMISSION CODE ORIGINAL REF. NO.

23. PRIOR AUTHORIZATION NUMBER

24. A DATE(S) OF SERVICE From MM DD YY To MM DD YY	B Place of Service	C Type of Service	D PROCEDURES, SERVICES, OR SUPPLIES (Explain Unusual Circumstances) CPT/HCPCS MODIFIER	E DIAGNOSIS CODE	F $ CHARGES	G DAYS OR UNITS	H EPSDT Family Plan	I EMG	J COB	K RESERVED FOR LOCAL USE
1										
2										
3										
4										
5										
6										

25. FEDERAL TAX I.D. NUMBER SSN EIN

26. PATIENT'S ACCOUNT NO.

27. ACCEPT ASSIGNMENT? (For govt. claims, see back) YES NO

28. TOTAL CHARGE $

29. AMOUNT PAID $

30. BALANCE DUE $

31. SIGNATURE OF PHYSICIAN OR SUPPLIER INCLUDING DEGREES OR CREDENTIALS (I certify that the statements on the reverse apply to this bill and are made a part thereof.)

SIGNED DATE

32. NAME AND ADDRESS OF FACILITY WHERE SERVICES WERE RENDERED (If other than home or office)

33. PHYSICIAN'S, SUPPLIER'S BILLING NAME, ADDRESS, ZIP CODE & PHONE #

PIN# GRP#

PHYSICIAN OR SUPPLIER INFORMATION

(APPROVED BY AMA COUNCIL ON MEDICAL SERVICE 8/88) ***PLEASE PRINT OR TYPE*** APPROVED OMB-0938-0008 FORM CMS-1500 (12-90), FORM RRB-1500, APPROVED OMB-1215-0055 FORM OWCP-1500, APPROVED OMB-0720-0001 (CHAMPUS)

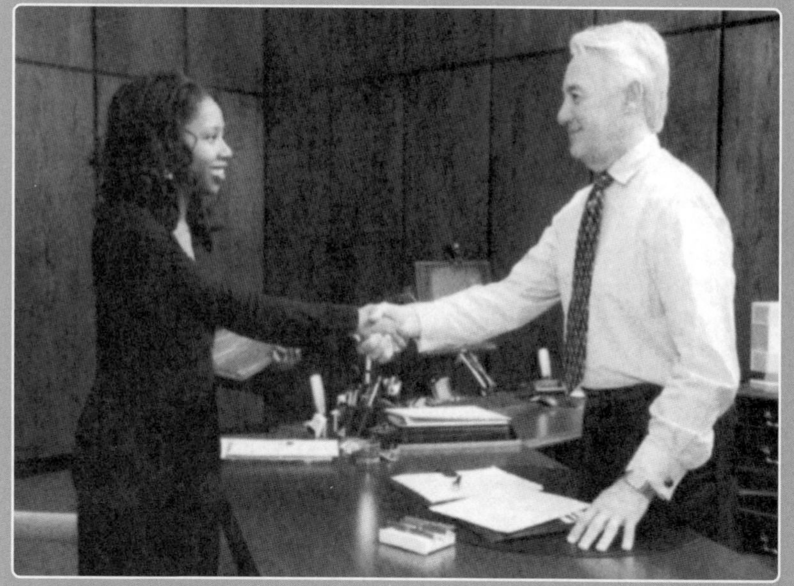

PART

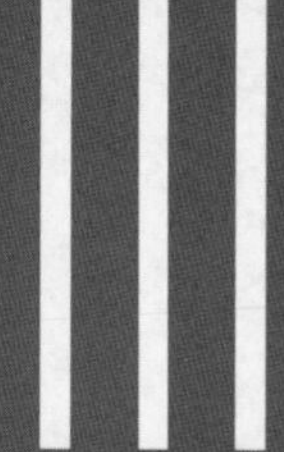

III Career Strategies

UNIT FOUR

Competing in the Job Market

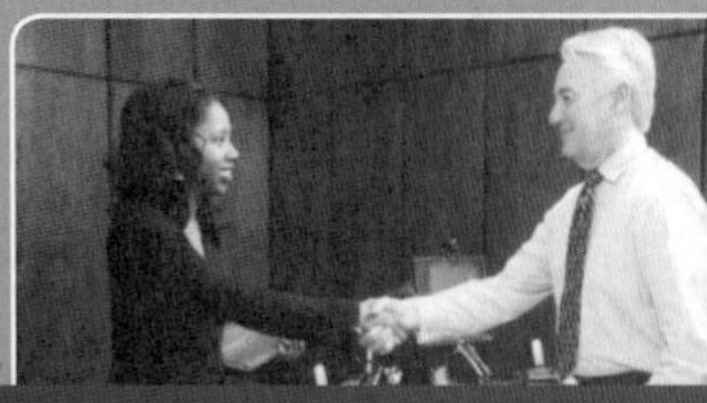

CHAPTER 16

Making the Transition: Student to Employee

Learning Outcomes

Cognitive Domain

1. Spell and define the key terms
2. Explain the purpose of the externship experience
3. Understand the importance of the evaluation process
4. List your professional responsibilities during externship
5. List personal and professional attributes necessary to ensure a successful externship
6. Determine your best career direction based on your skills and strengths
7. Identify the steps necessary to apply for the right position and be able to accomplish those steps
8. Draft an appropriate cover letter
9. List the steps and guidelines in completing an employment application
10. List guidelines for an effective interview that will lead to employment
11. Identify the steps that you need to take to ensure proper career advancement
12. Explain the process for recertification of medical assisting credentials
13. Describe the importance of membership in a professional organization
14. Recognize elements of fundamental writing skills
15. List and discuss legal and illegal interview questions
16. Discuss all levels of governmental legislation and regulation as they apply to medical assisting practice

Psychomotor Domain

1. Write a résumé to properly communicate skills and strengths (Procedure 16-1)
2. Compose professional/business letters

Affective Domain

1. Apply local, state, and federal health care legislation

ABHES Competencies

1. Comply with federal, state, and local health laws and regulations
2. Perform fundamental writing skills, including correct grammar, spelling, and formatting techniques when writing prescriptions, documenting medical records, etc.

Name: ______________________ Date: ____________ Grade: ____________

COG MULTIPLE CHOICE

1. Most externships range from:
   a. 160–240 hours a semester.
   b. 80–160 hours a semester.
   c. 200–240 hours a semester.
   d. 240–300 hours a semester.
   e. 260–300 hours a semester.
2. Preceptors are typically:
   a. physicians.
   b. nurses.
   c. graduate medical assistants.
   d. academic instructors.
   e. other students.
3. When responding to a newspaper advertisement, you should:
   a. mail your résumé and a portfolio.
   b. send your résumé by e-mail.
   c. phone right away to inquire about the job.
   d. follow the instructions in the advertisement.
   e. call to schedule an interview.
4. A CMA wishing to recertify must either retake the examination or complete:
   a. 60 hours of continuing education credits.
   b. 50 hours of continuing education credits.
   c. 100 hours of continuing education credits.
   d. 30 hours of continuing education credits.
   e. 75 hours of continuing education credits.
5. Two standard ways of listing experience on a résumé are:
   a. functional and chronological.
   b. functional and alphabetical.
   c. alphabetical and chronological.
   d. chronological and referential.
   e. referential and alphabetical.
6. During your externship, it is a good practice to arrive:
   a. a few minutes early.
   b. half an hour early.
   c. right on time.
   d. with enough time to beat traffic.
   e. as early as you can.
7. What is the appropriate length of a résumé?
   a. One page
   b. Two pages
   c. Three pages
   d. As long as it needs to be
   e. Check with the potential employer first
8. In addition to providing proof of general immunizations, what other vaccinations may be required before you begin your externship?
   a. Vaccination for strep throat
   b. Vaccination for cancer
   c. Vaccination for hepatitis B
   d. Vaccination for hepatitis C
   e. Vaccination for HIV
9. During your externship, you are expected to perform as:
   a. the student that you are; your preceptor will teach you the same skills as in the classroom.
   b. an experienced professional; your preceptor will expect you to perform every task perfectly.
   c. an entry-level employee; your preceptor will expect you to perform at the level of a new employee in the field.
   d. a patient; you have to see what it feels like to be on the receiving end of treatment.
   e. independently as possible; your preceptor will not have time to answer many questions.

10. Checking for telephone messages and arranging the day's appointments should be done:

a. during your lunch break.

b. at the close of the business day.

c. after the office has opened.

d. before the scheduled opening.

e. between patients.

11. Fingernails should be kept short and clean to avoid:

a. making your supervisor upset.

b. accidentally scratching or harming a patient.

c. transferring pathogens or ripping gloves.

d. getting nail polish chips in lab samples.

e. infecting sterile materials or surfaces.

12. Which document provides proof that tasks are performed and learning is taking place?

a. Timesheet

b. Journal

c. Survey

d. Evaluation

e. Personal interview

13. Which document is used to improve performance and services offered to students?

a. Timesheet

b. Journal

c. Survey

d. Evaluation

e. Personal interview

14. Membership in your professional allied health organization proves:

a. that you are an allied health student.

b. your level of professionalism and seriousness of purpose.

c. that you will become a medical professional in 2 years.

d. your willingness to network with other professionals.

e. your interest in the medical field.

15. Which question should you avoid asking during an interview?

a. Is there access to a 401(k) plan?

b. Is tuition reimbursement available?

c. How many weeks of vacation are available the first year?

d. Are uniforms or lab coats worn?

e. What are the responsibilities of this position?

16. If you decide to leave your job, it is a good idea to:

a. tell your employer the day before you plan to leave.

b. make sure your new job will pay more.

c. get contact information for all of the new friends you made.

d. finish all duties and tie up any loose ends.

e. criticize employees during an exit interview.

17. If you are having a problem performing your assigned job duties, it is best to:

a. volunteer for extra hours.

b. inform your preceptor and instructor.

c. ask for less challenging work.

d. ask for a different externship site.

e. switch your course of studies.

18. When anticipating calls from prospective employers, avoid:

a. leaving silly or cute messages on your answering machine.

b. telling family members or roommates that you are expecting important telephone calls.

c. keeping a pen near the telephone at all times.

d. checking messages on a regular basis.

e. calling them every day after submitting your résumé.

19. If bilingual applicants are encouraged to apply for a position you want, you should:

a. learn simple greetings and act as if you can speak several languages.

b. learn simple greetings and admit that you know a few words but are not fluent.

c. do nothing; being bilingual is not important.

d. avoid applying since you do not fluently speak another language.

e. learn how to answer possible interview questions in two different languages.

20. Being a lifelong learner is a must for all medical professionals because:

a. medical professionals have to recertify every 5 years.

b. medical professionals are widely respected.

c. changes in procedures, medical technologies, and legal issues occur frequently.

d. changes in medical technologies are decreasing the need for medical professionals.

e. medical professionals are required to change legal statutes once a year.

COG MATCHING

Grade: _______

Match the following key terms to their definitions.

Key Terms	Definitions
21. _____ externship	**a.** a teacher; one who gives direction, as in a technical matter
22. _____ networking	**b.** an educational course that allows the student to obtain hands-on experience
23. _____ portfolio	**c.** a system of personal and professional relationships through which to share information
24. _____ preceptor	**d.** a document summarizing an individual's work experience or professional qualifications
25. _____ résumé	**e.** a portable case containing documents

COG SHORT ANSWER

Grade: _______

26. What is the purpose of an externship?

____

____

____

____

27. List three responsibilities you will have during an externship.

a. ____

b. ____

c. ____

28. How will the site preceptor assist you in your externship?

____

____

____

____

29. List five traditional sources of information for job openings.

a. ______________________________

b. ______________________________

c. ______________________________

d. ______________________________

e. ______________________________

AFF PSY **REFLECTION** Grade: ________

30. Write a list of your strengths and weaknesses as discussed in the chapter. Critically evaluate what you are able to contribute to the job and address your weaknesses. How can you work with these weaknesses to make them strengths? Now evaluate what kind of medical assisting job would best work with what you are already good at and how you would like to continue to grow in your professional development. Identify for yourself what type of job would be ideal for you.

____

____

____

____

31. Practice interviewing with a fellow student. Make sure that you take turns asking questions so that you can both get to experience being on each side of the interview.

COG IDENTIFICATION

Grade: ________

32. Below are items that could be included on a résumé. Circle all that are appropriate.

a. contact information

b. race

c. relevant volunteer work

d. birth date

e. experience

f. picture of yourself

g. list of professional goals

h. education

i. credit history

j. references

k. date of high school graduation

Action Words

generates	ensures	implements and maintains	interviews	records	articulates
draws and collects	prepares	selects	measures	assists	composes

Choose a more accurate action word from the box to replace the words in bold.

33. Helps in examination and treatment of patients under the direction of a physician. ________

34. Talks to patients, **takes** vital signs (i.e., pulse rate, temperature, blood pressure, weight, and height), and **writes** information on patients' charts. ________

35. Gets blood samples from patients and prepare specimens for laboratory analysis. ________

36. Sets up treatment rooms for examination of patients. ________

37. Read each of the following tips for completing a job application. Circle all appropriate best practices for completing an application.

a. Read through the application completely before beginning.

b. Follow the instructions exactly.

c. In the line for wage or salary desired, write highest pay possible.

d. Answer every question. If the question does not apply to you, draw a line or write "N/A" so that the interviewer will know that you did not overlook the question.

e. Use your best cursive writing.

f. Highlight important information in red ink.

g. Ask for two applications. Use the first one for practice.

38. From the list of questions below, circle all that would be appropriate for a job applicant to ask a prospective employer.

a. What are the responsibilities of the position offered?

b. What is the benefit package? Is there access to a 401(k) plan or other retirement plan? Health insurance? Life insurance?

c. Is it acceptable to take 3 weeks off during the holiday season?

d. How does the facility feel about continuing education? Is time off offered to employees to upgrade their skills? Does the facility subsidize the expense?

e. Do I have to work with physicians who have bad attitudes?

f. How many potlucks and happy hours does this office usually have?

g. Is there a job performance or evaluation process?

COG EXPLANATION

Grade: ______

39. Explain what it means to be a lifelong learner

____

____

____

____

40. How can you prepare for the process of recertification?

____

____

____

____

41. List two professional organizations you could join while you are a student.

a. ____

b. ____

AFF WHAT WOULD YOU DO?

Grade: ________

42. The office manager at your extern site does not allow CMAs to give injections. At an office meeting, the employees ask her why not. Her reply is, "it is illegal." The employees tell her that it is not illegal for medical assistants to give injections in the state where you are. She is surprised to hear this and asks the group to prove it to her. Because you are a student and have skills in researching topics, they ask you to find the legislation and bring it to the office manager. Choose all appropriate actions from the list below.
    a. Go to the state Web site and search "general assembly."
    b. Search for the information on the AAMA Web site by entering key words, "CMA scope of practice."
    c. Search for the information in general statutes by entering key words, "health care legislation in [name of your state]."
    d. Search for the information by entering key words, "unlicensed health personnel" under *general assembly* in your state.
    e. Search for the information by entering key words, "practice of medicine."

43. While working as an extern at a family care provider, you encounter an older adult patient who is uncomfortable with the fact that you as a student are participating in her care. What would you say to help her feel more comfortable?

44. There are multiple gaps in your work history, and your interviewer asks you to explain why. One of the gaps is from relocation, and other gaps are from taking time off to evaluate what you wanted to be doing. How would you explain this to your interviewer?

45. During an interview, you are asked to explain why your grades were low last semester. How would you answer this question honestly while still speaking about yourself fairly and objectively?

COG TRUE OR FALSE?

Grade: _______

Determine whether the following statements are true or false. If false, explain why.

46. When you see dangerous practices, it is usually best to confront the employee first.

____

____

47. Problems encountered at an externship site are best handled by site employees who have experience working with the office manager.

____

____

48. It is a good idea to include hobbies and personal interests on your résumé.

____

____

49. It is a good idea to write a long and detailed cover letter.

____

____

AFF CASE STUDY FOR CRITICAL THINKING

Grade: _______

It is the first day of your medical assisting externship.

50. Your externship preceptor has said that you cannot receive permission to draw blood and perform other phlebotomy procedures. However, you know this is an area that you are required to complete. Circle all of the appropriate actions from the list below.

a. Tell your externship coordinator from your college at her next site visit.

b. Tell the preceptor that you must perform these tasks and leave.

c. Call your externship coordinator immediately.

d. Call a classmate and ask her what to do.

51. Your school will likely request that you fill out an evaluation form to determine if your externship site was effective for training. This helps the school decide if it is a good site for future externships. Review the list of questions below and circle all you should consider when filling out your site evaluation form on your externship.

    a. Was the overall experience positive or negative?

    b. Was my preceptor fun to be around?

    c. Did the office have a good cafeteria or break room?

    d. Were opportunities for learning abundant and freely offered or hard to obtain?

    e. Was my preceptor flexible about taking personal time during the day for phone calls and breaks?

    f. Were staff personnel open and caring or unwelcoming?

    g. Was the preceptor available and easily approachable or preoccupied and distant?

52. Choose all appropriate ways to dress for your externship from the list below.

    a. Burgundy and navy scrubs along with a set of bangle bracelets, your favorite gemstone rings, and a pair of comfortable white clogs.

    b. The required scrubs with a pair of clean white sneakers. Dreadlocks placed in a neat ponytail above the shoulders.

    c. The required uniform and a pair of dark walking shoes. Hair with the tips of a spiked mohawk dyed burgundy to match.

    d. The required uniform with white sneakers and college nametag.

    e. Street clothes with lab coat and required nametag.

    f. Long sleeves to cover the tattoo on your arm.

PORTFOLIO Grade: ________

Design and compile a portfolio to present at your upcoming job interviews. Refer to Chapter 16 for a list of possible contents of the portfolio. Remember, the purpose of a portfolio is to impress an interviewer. You have worked hard to earn your medical assisting certificate, diploma, or degree. This is your opportunity to show off your professional skills, abilities, and accomplishments.

PSY PROCEDURE 16-1 Writing a Résumé

Name: ____________________ Date: ________ Time: ________ Grade: ________

Equipment/Supplies: Word processor, paper, personal information

STANDARDS: Given the needed equipment and a place to work, the student will perform this skill with ______% accuracy in a total of ______ minutes. *(Your instructor will tell you what the percentage and time limits will be before you begin practicing.)*

KEY: 4 = Satisfactory 0 = Unsatisfactory NA = This step is not counted

PROCEDURE STEPS	SELF	PARTNER	INSTRUCTOR
1. At the top of the page, center your name, address, and phone numbers.	☐	☐	☐
2. List your education starting with the most current and working back. List graduation dates and areas of study. It is not necessary to go all the way back to elementary school.	☐	☐	☐
3. Using the chronological format, list your prior related work experience with dates, responsibilities, company, and supervisor's name.	☐	☐	☐
4. List any volunteer work with dates and places.	☐	☐	☐
5. List skills you possess, including those acquired in your program and on your externship.	☐	☐	☐
6. List any certifications or awards received.	☐	☐	☐
7. List any information relevant to a certain position (for example, competence in spreadsheet applications for a job in a patient billing department).	☐	☐	☐
8. After obtaining permission and/or notifying the people, prepare a list of references with their addresses and phone contact information.	☐	☐	☐
9. Carefully proofread the résumé for accuracy and typographical errors.	☐	☐	☐
10. Have someone else proofread the résumé for errors other than content.	☐	☐	☐
11. Print the résumé on high-quality paper.	☐	☐	☐
12. AFF You had only one job before finishing your medical assisting program. Should you try to "pad" your résumé by listing some anyway? Why or why not?	☐	☐	☐

____

____

____

____

CALCULATION

Total Possible Points: ______

Total Points Earned: ______ Multiplied by 100 = ______ Divided by Total Possible Points = ______ %

PASS ☐ **FAIL** ☐ **COMMENTS:**

Student's signature ______________________________ Date ______

Partner's signature ______________________________ Date ______

Instructor's signature ______________________________ Date ______

CHAPTER 17

Capstone Activities: Applying What You Have Learned

Working in a medical office means dealing with situations as they arise in a professional, nonjudgmental manner. Your education and training has provided you with the information and tools to give you administrative competence necessary to function in the medical office, but you must also use professional judgment and critical thinking when making decisions and interacting with patients, families, and staff. This chapter will provide opportunities for you to practice using professional judgment and critical thinking skills as would a practicing medical assistant in the physician office. Each section, containing documentation and active learning exercises, provides real-life scenarios followed by questions for you to think about and respond to according to directions from your instructor. Be sure to read carefully and, as usual, have fun!

COG PSY DOCUMENTATION

CHAPTER 1

Christopher Guest is waiting to see the physician, who has been called to the emergency room. You explain the situation to the patient, and he asks if you can perform his physical instead. You explain your scope of practice. Write a chart note to record the conversation.

CHAPTER 2

Your physician asks you to write a letter to Jean Mosley, a patient who has continued to be noncompliant. She wants to formally terminate the patient's care and refer her elsewhere. Write a note in the patient's chart documenting your actions.

CHAPTER 3

You are checking in a new patient who is obviously in acute pain. He is crying and pacing the floor. You take him to a private area to carry out the patient interview and help him complete his medical questionnaire. Write a note in the patient's chart documenting the fact that you assisted the patient with the questionnaire.

CHAPTER 4

Julia is an 8-year-old patient who has been diagnosed with juvenile diabetes. You supply the patient and her mother with educational materials about Julia's condition and how to manage her blood sugar. Write a chart note to document the conversation and actions.

CHAPTER 5

Megan O'Conner is a patient who was discharged from the hospital a few hours ago. She calls the office to report that she is now feeling woozy and nauseous. She thinks it might be a side effect of the pain medication she was given. Per your office protocol, she is advised to stop taking the medication, and you will have the doctor e-prescribe a different medication. Ms. O'Conner is obviously very upset. She is crying and says she just wants to go back to the hospital. You reassure her. Write a note about the conversation to be included in the chart.

CHAPTER 6

Mr. Sheffield did not show up for his appointment. You call him, and he says he forgot. You reschedule his appointment for the next day at 10:00 a.m. Write a note to document this in the chart.

CHAPTER 7

The physician asks you to write a note to a patient, Nancy Chesnutt, informing her of her normal lab results. Construct the note that would be included as a copy in the patient's chart.

CHAPTER 8

A patient requests release of his records to another physician. What documentation is necessary for this release? Write a note to document the release in the patient's chart.

CHAPTER 9

You receive an e-mail from Mr. Hagler saying that his medication is working out well and is not causing any side effects. He will be in for this appointment next Tuesday. How do you document this information in Mr. Hagler's medical record?

CHAPTER 10

During a routine visit, Carlos Delgado, a 55-year-old male, complains of tightness in his chest and nausea. He is short of breath and appears hypoxic. You notify the physician, and, when you return, Mr. Delgado is in respiratory arrest. EMS is called. The physician orders bag-to-mouth respirations with 6 L supplemental oxygen, which you provide. An AED is not available. After 5 minutes of artificial respirations, the patient enters full cardiac arrest, and the physician begins chest compressions. Five minutes later, EMS arrives to take the patient. Use the space below to record the incident in the chart.

CHAPTER 11

Ms. Bailey has a large balance, and she is in today to see the doctor. You have a conversation with her about her unpaid bill. She promises to send $50.00 on the fifth of each month beginning next month. Write a note to record this agreement for her financial record.

CHAPTER 12

Tonya Sushkin's insurance company paid $25.00 for an office visit on 7/14/13. Your physician is a participating provider for this company. Your initial charge was $75.00. Post the payment and adjustment on a blank daysheet. Ms. Sushkin's previous balance is $75.00.

CHAPTER 13

Laila Hildreath is a 4-year-old girl who needs to have tubes in her ears after failing conservative treatment for recurrent ear infections. Her father is a member of an HMO that requires preauthorization for surgery. You call the HMO and receive authorization for the in-patient procedure. You are given the following preauthorization number: 67034598 AB. Record your actions for the patient's financial record.

____

____

____

____

CHAPTER 14

The physician has asked you to write a letter to the insurance company requesting 1 more day for a patient to remain in the hospital due to the fact that she has an indwelling catheter.

____

____

____

____

CHAPTER 15

An 18-year-old woman is seen for a college physical. While being examined, she tells the physician's assistant that her boyfriend is abusive on occasion. The visit becomes predominantly counseling for the next 20 minutes of her 30-minute visit. How would you document this in the chart so that the visit can be coded accurately?

____

____

____

____

CHAPTER 16

You just completed an interview with the office manager of a large family practice. Write a thank you note to the interviewer.

____

____

____

____

PSY ACTIVE LEARNING

CHAPTER 1

Talk with a grandparent or another older adult, and ask him or her to tell you about a medical discovery that he or she remembers well. Create a "before and after" chart, explaining what life was like before the discovery, and the changes and benefits that came about after the discovery.

CHAPTER 2

Go to the Health and Human Services Web site, http://www.hhs.gov/ocr/privacy. What is the mission statement of the Office for Civil Rights regarding the HIPAA Privacy Rule?

CHAPTER 3

Do a Web search for "anger management techniques." Are there suggestions that could help you communicate with an angry patient? Record your findings. Cite Web sites used.

CHAPTER 4

Go to the Council on Aging's Web site, http://www.ncoa.org. Describe the plan included in the *Falls Free Coalition* outlined in the Safety of Seniors Act of 2008.

CHAPTER 5

Go the Americans With Disabilities Web site, http://www.usdoj.gov/crt/ada. Go to the Primer for Small Businesses. Who is covered by the ADA?

CHAPTER 6

Memorize the days of the week in Spanish. Recite them for your classmates.

CHAPTER 7

When writing, it is important to know your audience. The way you write for a physician is different from the way you write for a patient. In the case of a physician, you can assume he or she understands medical terminology, but this is not so of a patient. Do some Internet research to better understand the possible digestive side effects of a common medication like simvastatin (Zocor) or esomeprazole (Nexium). Then, write two letters discussing the side effects, one to a physician and one to a patient. Think about what you must do differently when writing to a patient.

CHAPTER 8

If you were opening a new medical facility, consider whether you would want staff members using abbreviations in patient records. Then create a list of acceptable abbreviations that may be used in your new facility. Then create a "Do Not Use" list for abbreviations that may be confusing and should not be included in records. Visit the Web site for the Joint Commission (http://www.jointcommission.org) and include all of those abbreviations in addition to five other abbreviations of your own choice.

CHAPTER 9

Go to WebMD (http://www.webmd.com). Scroll down to the Symptom Checker. Think back to your last illness or pick an illness and answer the questions about the symptoms. What do you have?

CHAPTER 10

Prepare a list of emergency contacts in the area, including the contact information of local hospitals, poison control centers, and emergency medical services.

CHAPTER 11

Call two collection agencies in your local area. Compare services and fees. Record your findings.

CHAPTER 12

Research the banking services offered by your local bank. Gather brochures outlining the services. Share with classmates to compare services.

CHAPTER 13

When will/did ICD-10 CM codes go into effect? Search http://www.aapc.com/ICD-10 for the answer.

CHAPTER 14

Find the ICD-9-CM codes for the following diseases:

a. Acute gastric ulcer with hemorrhage and perforation without obstruction____________________

b. Meningococcal pericardiitis____________________

c. Impetigo____________________

d. Benign essentiahypertension____________________

CHAPTER 15

Research the subject of Current Procedural Coding. Write a paragraph describing the origin of the CPT codes. What was the original purpose of CPT coding?

CHAPTER 16

Do an Internet search of medical assisting job opportunities in your area. Now broaden your search to check jobs in any large metropolitan area. What are the differences and similarities in your local opportunities and those in the other city?